HUGH ALDERSEY-WILLIAMS is a writer and curator with interests ranging from science to architecture and design. His prolific career as a freelance journalist included a five-year stint as the design critic of the *New Statesman*. He is the author of *Periodic Tales: The Curious Lives of the Elements* ˥d *Anatomies: The Human Body, Its Parts and the Stories They Tell*. He lives with his family in Norfolk and has been an unreasoning Thomas Browne fan for many years.

'Engaging and thoughtful…Like some of the most compelling biographers, Aldersey-Williams partly inhabits his subject. [It is] less like a biography, more like a mental inhabitation' *Literary Review*

'This is not a conventional biography. It is more a conversation with an old friend. An engaging and often funny book' *Economist*

'Charming' *Sunday Telegraph*

The
Adventures
of
Sir Thomas Browne
in the 21st Century

HUGH ALDERSEY-WILLIAMS

GRANTA

941.06092

Granta Publications, 12 Addison Avenue, London, W11 4QR

First published in Great Britain by Granta Books 2015
This paperback edition published by Granta Books 2015

A CIP catalogue record for this book is available from the British Library

9 8 7 6 5 4 3 2 1

ISBN 978 1 84708 902 1 (paperback)
ISBN 978 1 84708 901 4 (ebook)

www.grantabooks.com

Designed and typeset in Adobe Caslon Pro by Lindsay Nash

Printed and bound by CPI Group (UK) Ltd, Croydon, CR0 4YY

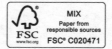

To Moira
who understood all along

Contents

Prologue

WHAT WAS HE thinking?

What was he thinking that morning in 1662 as he set out from the spring assizes at Bury St Edmunds towards his home in the city of Norwich? It was a full day's ride in fair conditions, and all the more arduous in this season when the road was liable to be churned to mud or sheathed in ice. He would have many hours to reflect, if he chose, on what he had said and its consequences.

A few days before, his words had done nothing to prevent two women from being sent to their deaths.

He had been present at a trial of two witches. Six girls and an infant boy, all of Lowestoft in Suffolk, were said to have been bewitched. The girls were a mute presence in the court, perhaps intimidated by the formality of the proceedings, or too scarred by their experience to speak up. Parents gave zealous testimony on their behalf. Each of the children had suffered fits and bouts of lameness and was said to have vomited up pins and nails. They had accused two widows, Amy Denny and Rose Cullender, of afflicting them. Amy Denny was the main culprit. She was a quarrelsome old woman, well known to the townspeople of Lowestoft, occasionally used by some of the parents for childcare, but had been put in the stocks the previous year by one of them for some unrecorded misdemeanour. Rose Cullender seems to have had less direct association with the children, and may simply have been fingered as another awkward old crone who would add weight to claims of witchcraft. The accused women were present in the courtroom, with Amy in particular shouting out in violent rebuttal of the denunciations made against her.

His name was Thomas Browne, and he was a physician by profession, trained at the best European schools of anatomy and medicine. He was also a philosopher and writer, a coiner of words, a Christian moralist, a naturalist, an antiquarian, an experimenter and a myth-buster. Called before the Bury assize as 'a Person of great knowledge', he was asked by the three serjeants-at-law for his opinion of the evidence they had heard.

What he said next was brief and was not in itself pivotal to the verdict handed down, but it can only have helped send the women on their way to the gallows. Browne recounted news of a 'Great Discovery of Witches' lately in Denmark, who had stuck pins into 'Afflicted Persons' in just the same way that Denny and Cullender were accused of doing. He offered his physician's opinion that the fits and other symptoms exhibited by the children were natural. Almost gratuitously, it seems, he then added the thought that this very naturalness was evidence of the 'subtilty' of the devil, who was controlling the witches' actions.

The serjeants had been divided before Browne spoke, uncertain they had heard enough to convict the women. Now his casual anecdote, which might have been taken as hearsay but for his learned reputation, made them think again. As for Browne, duty done, he probably did not remain in Bury for long after the trial to see the women hanged. He had patients waiting to see him in Norwich.

I decide to pursue Thomas Browne on his journey from Bury to Norwich.

The Shire Hall where the 1662 assizes were held no longer stands. The site where Honey Hill runs down to the watermeadows of the rivers Lark and Linnet has been redeveloped with modern council offices. But other parts of the town have changed little, and it is obvious what route Browne would have taken. In order to approximate the scale and texture of Browne's journey, to match its pace and to be able to see what Browne would have seen, I go by bicycle. I want time to think about what was going through Browne's head.

I am grateful for a mild and dry day as I set off, 350 years to the month after Browne. Weather records for 1662 show the spring to have been kind that year too, and perhaps in the end Browne made good speed. I pedal up Honey Hill, and turn right at the vast parish church of St Mary's to head down the broad sweep of Angel Hill past the extensive complex of St Edmund's Abbey, much of it as Browne would have seen it, in ruins since the dissolution of the monasteries, its stones ransacked for godless new buildings. I skirt the great marketplace where Denny and Cullender were briefly imprisoned before they were hanged, and turn right again onto Eastgate, crossing over the river past the old Edward VI grammar school. Then it's up the long, slow incline onto the exposed road east.

To the shepherd or woodsman who chanced to see him pass by, Browne would not have cut an imposing figure. He was in his fifties, of slight build and habitually plainly dressed for a man of his standing. The bystander would have gleaned nothing from this unpromising exterior about the man's remarkable heart and mind. Browne was loved by his patients, who admired his readiness to treat rich and poor, Catholic and Protestant alike. He was more widely renowned, too, as the author of philosophical essays. The earliest of these contentiously sought to reconcile his rationalism as a physician with his Christian faith. Others, more in the spirit of the age, discuss antiquities and the meaning of death or the significance of pattern and number in nature. His greatest and most popular work, though, was a vast catalogue of 'vulgar errors', seven volumes of foolish common beliefs of the seventeenth century, each in turn set out and then learnedly, scientifically, gently and humorously debunked.

He could write this humane and sceptical work, and yet he believed in witches. He freely gave his opinion on the existence of witches before and after the incident at Bury. But of the trial itself, he seems to have had no further thought. Was it for him simply a matter of course? Was it an episode to forget?

I settle to a steady pace as I cycle through the ancient villages of Ixworth and Stanton and the Rickinghalls Inferior and Superior, and then run across the heaths and commons of Wortham and Palgrave to skirt the marshes south of Diss. The blackthorn is coming out. Perhaps Browne was able to immerse himself in the details of awakening life as

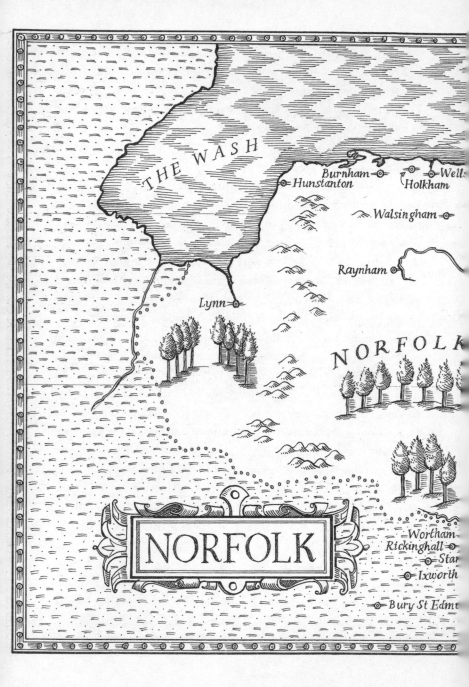

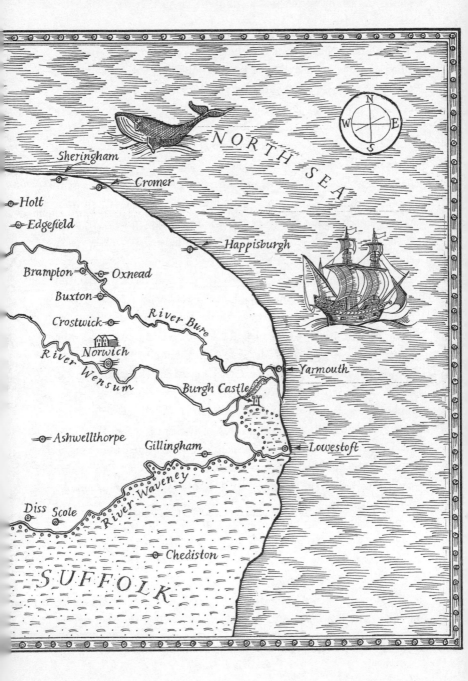

NORTH SEA

Sheringham

Cromer

Holt

Edgefield

Happisburgh

Brampton

Oxnead

Buxton

Crostwick

River Bure

Norwich

River Wensum

Yarmouth

Burgh Castle

Ashwellthorpe

Gillingham

Lowestoft

River Waveney

Diss

Scole

Chediston

SUFFOLK

he rode on. Perhaps his horse flushed up skylarks from the Breckland scrub and he caught the scent of herbs familiar from his own physic garden. On my journey, though, I see mainly flattened drinks bottles, hubcaps in the hedgerows, and dead pigeons batted aside by the speeding traffic.

He may have smiled when he reached the Dolphin Inn at Wortham. At the time he was in the middle of gathering observations that would go towards the compilation of *Notes and Letters on the Natural History of Norfolk*, a catalogue of the birds and fishes found in the county. He offers a clear description of the common dolphin, so as to distinguish it from the porpoise. The animal has a 'very good taste to most palates', he adds.

The inn has a forlorn air that its pink paint is unable to lift. A young couple nurse their ciders, at a loss for conversation at its single picnic table on the green. Its sign is simple gold lettering on black with a token squiggle of ornamentation. Perhaps there was once a painting of a dolphin, not as accurate as that given by the French naturalist Rondelet, which Browne took as his guide for identification, more likely the stylized version of heraldry, a leaping arch of muscle. Browne devotes an entire volume of *Pseudodoxia Epidemica* to 'things questionable as they are commonly described in Pictures', and one of his subjects is the dolphin. He worries that people will think they actually occur in nature as they are habitually depicted, in this scoliotic way rather than lithe and flexible of spine. Such an argument might seem pedantic, like the person today who points out that a cartoon figure is unrealistic, but it matters in an age when uncritical belief in images frequently triumphs over observation and reason.

Occasionally, amid the prairie-like fields, there are orchards of budding apple trees, and I look over to see if they are arranged in the manner celebrated by Browne in his essay on horticulture, *The Garden of Cyrus*. Browne was captivated by the ancient custom of planting orchards in overlapping quincunxes, modules of five trees set out in an X like the five dots on a die. The essay revels in the subtitle *The Quincunciall, Lozenge, or Net-work Plantations of the Ancients, Artificially,*

Naturally, Mystically Considered. It is a work of skilled scientific obser-vation rooted in the East Anglian landscape, but also a disquisition of quite startling breadth, taking into its ambit the origins of gardens, the shapes of various crosses, ornament in classical architecture and the art of the lapidary. Holding it all loosely together is the number five, the generator of so many patterns and repetitions in nature.

I recall the moment when Thomas Browne invaded my life. It happened when I was writing a book about the discovery in 1985 of a new form of carbon called buckminsterfullerene. This form of the element has atoms bonded to one another in such a way as to form a curved pattern of hexagons and pentagons like the stitching on the surface of a soccer ball. The pentagons that punctuate the surface of the buckminsterfullerene molecule would make a fine addition to Browne's miscellany of the five-fold.

As I travel on, I cannot help seeing Browne's mysterious signs of natural order everywhere I look. They are visible in fallen pine cones and the wind-dried heads of teasels, and in the 'catkins, or pendulous excres-cencies of severall Trees, of Wallnuts, Alders and Hazels, which hanging all the Winter, and maintaining their Net-worke close, by the expansion thereof are the early foretellers of the Spring'. I think of the starfish and viruses that also exhibit five-fold symmetry. It is clear that this number really does have a special place in nature. It is even strangely evident in the man-made world, I realize. Most of the hubcaps in the hedges are perforated with five holes and have the same pentagonal symmetry as Browne's flowers and seeds.

The words of the trial echo through my head. I see that in his own mind, if not in the view of the judge and complainants determined to return a guilty verdict, Browne's contribution was carefully equivocal. He had called the children's affliction natural, and had added that their malady was merely heightened by the agency of the devil. He had never said they were caused directly by witches, nor that those witches were the women in the court. Such equivocation is characteristic of Browne and marks him apart from most men of his time. He could always see both sides of the argument. Sometimes, this was a virtue – it was not easy to keep a level head and maintain an attitude of tolerance during the English Civil War. At other times, he is equivocal to a fault, marshalling the arguments for and against some dubious phenomenon in nature or metaphysical nicety with the greatest eloquence, yet never coming down on one side himself.

Did he feel that his medical view that the children's suffering could be regarded as entirely natural had been given due weight? Or did he regret that it had been swept aside by more melodramatic testimony, by the impassioned pleas of the parents, by the pitiful appearance of the silent children, and by his own careless afterthought about the Danish case? Did he consider what he could have said that might have led to a more humane outcome? Did it ever occur to him to suggest that a belief in witches, while still perfectly respectable and perfectly tenable in 1662, was actually rather old fashioned, and in fact well on the way to becoming superstition, another 'vulgar error'?

Of course, we cannot know. Indeed, we cannot even be sure exactly what Browne said in court. The only record of the trial was made twenty years later. We cannot be sure, therefore, that its account of Browne's evidence is accurate or complete, just as we cannot be sure that the judge was as impartial as he is made to appear, or that the women really were given the opportunity to 'confess'.

I have not withheld facts for the sake of spinning out this yarn. I would really like to know what Browne said and thought – about the case, about the medical and bedevilled condition of the defendants, about witches in general, and for that matter about the plaintiffs and their motives. But the suspect nature of the trial record, and the absence of any discussion in Browne's own hand, forces me to reflect on our own time. It makes me realize we cannot be sure even of what goes on in today's criminal justice proceedings and inquiries into strange practices. All records, however authoritative, are necessarily incomplete and approximate. The words in print do not represent exactly what was said and what was said never represents exactly what was meant or taken as meant.

How Browne would have smiled at my difficulty. Uncertainty was his stock in trade, and judging between uncertainty and unknowability his unique talent. This readiness to mark out a realm for the mysterious no doubt stems from a proper God-fearing humility, but I think it also shows that Browne has identified an arena for delight. He recognizes, as many, especially scientists, do not, that description is not the key to understanding all. Words cannot transmit the truth; in fact, they put layers between us and the truth. Browne's genius was not only to accept this, but also to revel in it, finding in language not a constricting cage but a bird ready to take flight.

At Scole I turn northward and cross the River Waveney into Norfolk. Still scarcely halfway to Norwich, my legs ache and my knuckles are chilled. I note with longing the imposing brick inn at Scole, new in Browne's day, where he may have rested for the night.

A kingfisher flashes by. One of the odder beliefs that Browne addressed in his catalogue of 'vulgar errors', *Pseudodoxia Epidemica*, was that a dead kingfisher makes a good weathervane. He calls it a strange opinion, but notes that it was nevertheless a living custom. Then he does a very Brownean thing: he tries it for himself. He procures a dead kingfisher, rigs it up, and finds ... that it doesn't work. 'As for experiment,' he reports, 'we cannot make it out by any we have attempted; for if a single King-fisher be hanged up with untwisted silk in an open room, and where the air is free, it observes not a constant respect unto the mouth of the wind, but variously converting, doth seldom breast it right.' Not convinced? Well, then he goes on to suspend two of the unfortunate birds and finds that as often as not they point in opposite directions.

It seems that Browne was not present at the stage in the trial at which the afflicted children were brought into contact with the accused women to see what effect they truly exerted. Here, surely, he would have been given pause for thought. For this direct empirical evidence flatly contradicted the idea that Denny and Cullender had any unique powers. Yet, predictably enough, even this further revelation was to be twisted into further evidence for bewitching.

At length, after cresting a number of hills that might have seemed gentle at the start of my ride, I see the spire of Norwich cathedral pricking the horizon ahead of me. I am relieved that my journey is nearly over. Thomas Browne, too, must have felt glad to be nearing home at last, and may have rejoiced for more a particular reason than I at the appearance of this symbol.

The Christian faith was a central and considered feature of Browne's life. In one way, it entirely explains and excuses his belief in witches. The women's indictment at the assize formally invoked the devil, and belief in the devil was a necessary concomitant of belief in God. He did not need to have seen a witch, or to see witchcraft being performed, in order to believe in witches. They were an article of faith.

However, in the end this is not enough. Browne is in fact surprisingly selective when it comes to what he believes in the Christian story. In his *Religio Medici* of 1643, the essay in which he seeks to square his scientific rationality with his faith, he finds numerous points of disagreement. He does not believe in the literal truth of Noah's flood, for example, citing the existence of American species not described in the Bible in his refutation. His scepticism in other matters leads us to wish he had been equally sceptical about the truth of witches. Notwithstanding the presence of the two women in the court, did Browne actually ever see a witch? For remember that although he had spoken of witches, and clearly indicated his personal belief in their existence, he does not appear to have made any comment on the demonic status of the accused. Were his skills of scientific observation and experiment ever tested in this way? How would he tell a witch if he did see one? He saw 'bewitched' behaviour, but he never describes having seen a witch.

This doesn't matter, though. The girls in the courtroom had clearly been bewitched, and they had accused Denny and Cullender of the crime, and that was pretty much an end of it. Browne may simply have left Bury satisfied to know that justice had been done and that he had done his duty by the Church and by the state – to king and country, as he might have reflected with quiet satisfaction in these months following the restoration of the monarchy. Although he personally never doubted the existence of witches, he was nevertheless quite capable of doubting the legitimacy of accusations of witchcraft. But on this crucial occasion he had not found it necessary to do so.

Thomas Browne is my obsession. He stands at the gates of modern science and yet remains happily in thrall to the ancient world and its mysteries, and he writes in intense colours about both of them. He is, I believe, insufficiently known and unjustly neglected. As a literary figure, he is now less well known than his admirers, who include Samuel Johnson, Coleridge, Melville, Poe, Emerson and Dickinson, Jorge Luis Borges, and, in this century, W. G. Sebald and Javier Marías. This is not, admittedly, a roll call of the most read – it is not Dickens, Hemingway, J. K. Rowling – but it does reveal some powerful affinities. 'Few people love the writings of Sir Thomas Browne,' said Virginia Woolf, 'but those who do are of the salt of the Earth.' Who would not want to join this elite?

His essays are one of the glories of the English language, but he also changed the way we use it. He invented essential words such as *medical*, as well as *precarious* and *insecurity* and *incontrovertible* and *hallucination*, words that speak with new precision of the coming struggle to distinguish the real from the imagined and the true from the doubtful. Was the existence of witches as incontrovertible as Browne thought? Or were the children at the Bury trial merely the victims or perpetrators of a kind of mass hallucination?

As a scientist, Browne is still less favoured. His investigations were too marginal – he was never a fellow of the new Royal Society – and too much directed towards building his own literary edifice. Among scientists today, the evolutionary theorist and writer Stephen Jay Gould was an admirer, but Richard Dawkins certainly is not – he can't tolerate Browne's readiness to believe in things that can't be shown. And that too is perhaps a clue as to why we should like Browne more.

Since I came across him, while writing about the symmetrical buckminsterfullerene, Browne has never quite left me. I find he resurfaces at moments that have nothing in common except their unpredictability. He has haunted me, and now, I have decided, it is my turn to haunt him. I will try to show why Browne means so much to me and why he should mean more to all of us.

This is not so much an attempt to piece together a biography of a forgotten master of English literature and science. His life is poorly documented, and in the end, it is his own writing that remains the best place to look if we are to reveal his life of tolerance, humour, serenity and untiring curiosity.

I want to do something a little different. These qualities of Browne's are qualities we need in greater abundance today. Browne's preoccupations – how to disabuse the credulous of their foolish beliefs, the meaning of order in nature, how to achieve a reconciliation between science and religion, how to think about death and life – are our preoccupations. In the twenty-first century, they are often the focus of dogmatic debate that generates heat but little light. Thomas Browne's spirit could teach us how to think more generously about these things. I want to transport that spirit into our present, which is beset with its own conflicts and areas of darkness no less than Browne's seventeenth century.

As I rest my bike at last against the wall of the sandwich shop that now occupies the site of Browne's house just off the Market Place in Norwich, I feel strongly that Thomas Browne is a sympathetic subject. I love the way his mind works and I love his writing. I feel I would like to have known him. I would have submitted gladly to his professional ministrations, and listened keenly as he distracted me with his latest musings. And yet he presents a problem, too. I cannot easily condone his actions at the Bury assize, neither from the standpoint of the present, nor even, I believe, from that of his own time. If Browne is to be the hero of my book, he is off to a poor start. If he is a scientist, why is he sometimes so infuriatingly unscientific? If he is a man of faith, why does he plainly doubt so much? And if he is, as he implies in *Religio Medici* he might like to be thought, a 'champion for truth', then what is truth?

Introduction

'Tis too late to be ambitious'

Urne-Buriall

W E KNOW WHAT Browne looked like. A few pictures were made
of him during his lifetime, paintings as well as engravings
to appear in his published works. The best of them is a small double
portrait of him with his wife, Dorothy, attributed to Joan Carlile, in the
collection of the National Portrait Gallery. A grimy portrait of Thomas
alone, possibly copied from it, hangs in St Peter Mancroft, the parish
church in Norwich where Browne worshipped. When it came up for
sale in the twentieth century, it was optimistically billed as a 'Picture
of Charles I and his Queen by Vandyck', but it is all the more striking
for its true authorship. Carlile was one of the first women in England
to paint professionally. It is not known whether her sex was a reason in
itself for the Brownes to award the commission; the artist was probably
found via a mutual friend.

She shows the Brownes looking at us, but turned three quarters
towards each other. They seem a little uncomfortable, as if they have
been asked to stand unnaturally close together by the artist. The painting was done when Browne was perhaps forty years old and Dorothy
was in her mid-twenties. We see a happily married couple in the prime
of life. It is the only evidence of Dorothy's appearance: she looks like a
china doll. A fringe of fair hair under her lace cap, and a curl of amusement on her lips. She is wearing a blue dress (over time, it has faded
almost to white) with a lace collar and dark jewels pendant at her breast.
Thomas's head seems likewise large in proportion to a body that is
further diminished by its disappearance into the black oil background.
His cheeks have a healthy blush. Thin hair covers his scalp and hangs in

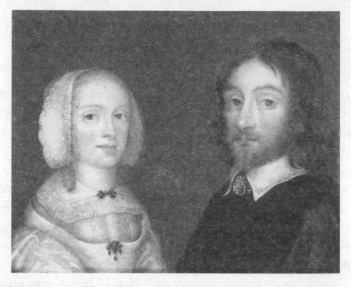

lank, loose curls. His boldly arced eyebrows, his moustache and beard have a reddish tinge. His gaze, from vast limpid eyes, is direct and a little sorrowful. He is dressed according to his usual fashion in plain but well-made dark clothes with only the tassels and turn-down collar of a white shirt showing at the neck.

One other item can provide solid evidence of Browne's likeness: his skull, which also resides at St Peter Mancroft in the form of a plaster cast. Browne's original burial place in this church was under the chancel where there is a plaque commemorating him. But the lid of his coffin was broken during a later interment in 1840. 'The accidental circumstance afforded an opportunity of inspecting the remains,' the *Norwich Chronicle* reported with barely hidden glee.

The bones of the skeleton were found to be in good preservation, particularly those of the skull. The brain was considerable in quantity but changed to a state of adipocere – resembling ointment of a dark brown hue. The hair of the beard remained profuse and perfect, though the flesh of the face, as well as of every other part, was totally gone. With respect to the conformation of the head, we are informed that the forehead was remarkably low, but the back of the cranium exhibited an unusual degree of depth and capaciousness.

In order to appreciate this story properly, it is necessary to know that adipocere, or 'grave wax', a soap-like substance formed by the decomposition of fat tissue, was first described by Browne himself upon observing a body that had lain buried in damp ground for some ten years. It can provide useful evidence in the forensic investigation of corpses today.

Following the disturbance, Browne's bones were to be reburied. However, a local surgeon, Edward Lubbock, took the skull – as a memento of an illustrious forebear rather than as a teaching specimen, one hopes – and it duly passed into the exhibition collection of the Norfolk and Norwich Hospital when he died.

In 1893, the vicar of St Peter Mancroft, prompted by an embarrassing mention of its disappearance in the London newspapers, wrote to ask for the skull back. 'We should any of us be shocked if the grave of our parents were rifled, and any part of their trusted remains exhibited in a museum. I cannot say the lapse of time in this case makes any difference.' The vicar deployed the full emotional armoury, referring darkly to the 'sacrilegious act' of the theft, and suggesting that Browne himself had been 'extremely anxious that his body should after death be treated with due reverence'. The hospital stonewalled. Privately, the churchmen began to doubt the authenticity of the object they were claiming. 'We don't know whether it really is his or somebody's else, or indeed where it came from,' the vicar wrote to his canon. The relic was only returned nearly thirty years later following the appointment of a more conciliatory secretary of the hospital.

Browne would have been resigned to the indignities his remains have undergone. In the dedication of *Urne-Buriall* to an old college friend, he wrote blithely: 'who knows the fate of his bones, or how often he is to be buried? Who hath the Oracle of his ashes, or whether they are to be scattered?' The returned skull was reinterred with due ceremony and to the satisfaction of all parties in July 1922. The parish register records the occasion: in the column provided for the age of the deceased is written the number 317.

Before this was done, however, the cast was made by the Royal College of Surgeons of England. I make an arrangement to see it. The cranium is remarkably smooth and of even convexity, without bumps or indentations. The mandible is separate, sans teeth and broken in three pieces. Both parts are weathered, though whether the cast has aged or the damage is faithfully imprinted from the original skull I cannot tell. I'd like to think of it as something more, but it seems to me just the

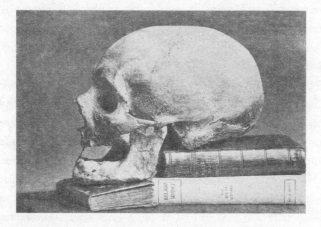

cast of an average skull; it is, as one nineteenth-century church official argued to the hospital, 'an ordinary one, of no scientific merit'. For the record, I ask the sacristan if I may measure it. It seems a Brownean thing to do. According to my makeshift calipers, Browne's head was 14.7 centimetres wide measured to the full extent of the parietal bones. From the crown of the head to the bottom of the lug below the rear of the cheekbone, known to physicians as the mastoid process, is 14.0 centimetres, and from the back of the head to the tip of the nasal bone is 22.2 centimetres. Since, as Browne wrote, 'the dimensions of the head measure the whole body', my measurements confirm that he was not a large man.

He would say that his physical body was the least of him. He would direct us to his written works: *Religio Medici*, *Pseudodoxia Epidemica*, *The Garden of Cyrus*, *Urne-Buriall* and others. Their titles seem wilfully obscure, and they have been for a long time little read. But their contents need not be found obscure at all.

Religio Medici, his first published work, is a confession, the highly personal exploration of a professional man in his thirties as he struggles to reconcile his devout but conventional Christian faith with his profession as a modern physician and natural philosopher. It was difficult material at a difficult time. He wrote it shortly before the outbreak of the English Civil War, and not long after publication it was placed on the papal index of prohibited books. The way in which he resolves for himself the counter-forces of religion and science has a poise that eludes many of those still seeking to square the two today.

His major work is *Pseudodoxia Epidemica*, a catalogue of 'vulgar errors', of the kind of things that uneducated people commonly believed in seventeenth-century England. If an orthodoxy is something that we correctly believe, then a pseudodoxy is something incorrectly held as fact. And an 'epidemic pseudodoxy' is something incorrectly held as fact by many. Browne debunks these foolish beliefs – that chameleons live only on air, that a diamond will dissolve in goat's blood – one by one, subdividing them into vast categories, errors mineral, vegetable and animal, errors to do with man, errors seen in pictures, errors in geography and history, and errors in scripture. Or, sometimes he doesn't. On the question of whether gold imbibed is a useful medicine, he equivocates; he cannot see what medical effect it might have, but he cannot be sure it has none. On the popular practice among pregnant women of holding a stone to the belly to ease labour pains, Browne doubts the purported source of these stones – they were said to come from eagles' nests – but can see no medical harm in the custom. If it works for you, he says in effect, then I won't stop you.

His method is rhetorical and scientific by turns. Often, he appeals to classical authority – you may think it is this, but Aristotle, or Pliny, or

Galen, long ago said it was that. Other times, he persuades us by logical argument. Occasionally, he illuminates the truth of some mysterious natural phenomenon with reference to scientific knowledge that he has acquired during his studies on the continent, information almost sure to be new to his English readers. Most appealing of all, he now and then seeks to convince us that some widely held opinion is an error by describing the results of his own little experiment. He knows a dead kingfisher does not make a good weathervane; he has tried it.

The Garden of Cyrus and *Urne-Buriall* might seem on first sight to be less considerable works. The former deals with aspects of form and geometry in nature, while the latter is an essay prompted by the unearthing of some Romano-British funerary relics. They make a literary diptych of the natural environment – what grows above the ground, and what decays beneath it – and man's place in its mysterious cycles. They display Browne's mature style as a writer. His long, rolling sentences compel admiration like complex natural phenomena, shells or orchids, say, or waves breaking languorously on a beach. But they also demonstrate the emergent methods of the botanist and the archaeologist.

In *Pseudodoxia Epidemica* he is a supreme sceptic. He is sceptical about everything, and he teaches us to how to be so too. Today, it might seem that his work is done. At every turn, there is a sceptic, loudly doubting the efficacy of alternative medicine, or denying the existence of God. Nor are the sceptics all on the 'side' of science. There are also sceptics who doubt the validity of scientific evidence for climate change or the truth of pharmaceutical manufacturers' claims for their products. But Browne's scepticism is different; he is sceptical but also humane. Even when he wishes to give an exceptionally loopy idea short shrift, his patience and good humour shine through. He agrees that various minerals have an effect on the body, for example, but 'that an Amethyst prevents inebriation...we are yet, I confess, to believe, and in that infidelity are likely to end our days'. If his humour is occasionally sardonic – the notion that every plant should be named after the disease it cures he reckons as 'A way more likely to multiply

Empericks [medical charlatans] then Herbalists' – it is at no person's direct expense. Not only that, he is able to empathize with proponent and opponent alike.

It is not the substance of the topics that Browne deals with but the way he deals with them that we need to recapture today: his civility, his tolerance, his good humour, his wit, and his sheer style. He is almost unfailingly forgiving of those with whom he disagrees, whether they follow religions or creeds other than his own, whether they disagree with him on matters of science and medicine, or whether they are simply ignorant (and we are almost all ignorant alongside Sir Thomas). He handles his imagined readers with kindness and generosity, treating them to little jokes and beautiful turns of phrase, and if these fall on deaf ears, it is no matter, for the thrust of his argument will not have been made to depend upon these niceties.

Because he belongs so resolutely to his time, and because, for some, his subject matter is arcane and occasionally even distasteful, he has been labelled for his pains as cheerless, melancholy and quaint. But he is genuinely entertaining in all these works. He is constantly stimulating, perceptive, unexpected. He is often prescient – often, but not always; sometimes he is happy to remain well behind the times. And he is occasionally downright funny – which is quite a trick given the seriousness of his times and the prodigality of his topics.

These are the works of a man finding time to write about whatever curious thing he has seen in between a doctor's rounds. He does not lose sight of the fact, and nor should we, that his day job was, as he quips in the introduction to *Urne-Buriall*, 'to keep men out of their Urnes'.

There is one thing that connects Browne with his texts, his corporeal body with his body of work, and that is his handwriting. The Norfolk Record Office holds a little of Browne's correspondence (much more is in the British Library). Searching through, I am excited to find also a rare manuscript copy of *Religio Medici*. The little book is bound in calf-skin and comprises 186 pages with about twenty-five hand-ruled lines to a page. There are red rules top and bottom and fainter ones making left and right margins. The text is inscribed neatly inside these boxes, each line justified by eye. Every straight stroke of the pen has a slight ogee and a subtle shift of line thickness, so that it looks like a natural organism trapped on the page rather than an artificial mark.

But I learn later that this is not Browne's hand, merely that of an unknown scribe. His actual letters display a prose less burnished than his famous essays and a script that is here attractive and tidy, here on the edge of ragged, perhaps according to how familiar he is with his correspondent. A slight italic tells me he was right-handed. The ascenders of his d's loop back spirally; y's slice emphatically downward; th's are accelerated into lightning zigzags. A majuscule J (in 'Inigo Jones') is finely formed with two passes of the nib. The odd character is finished off with a flourish that sweeps below the line of the text and thickens into a scimitar blade. Sometimes Browne's pen does not leave the paper from one word to the next. The inking – now appearing a dark coffee-brown in colour – is so even that it is often impossible to tell when he dips his pen. There are no blots and only a few short crossings-out. Even in old age, his writing remains fluent. The manuscript of *Repertorium*, written around 1680, an inventory of tombs at Norwich Cathedral, a building which he had seen ransacked during the Commonwealth, is less controlled and more rapid, but still quite legible.

It is writers more than scientists who have tended to champion Browne. His delirious style sees to that. But not all the literary greats line up to praise him; not even very many do so. Those who do are a particular selection, and it is a particular Browne that they admire.

It is no surprise that Samuel Johnson should have chosen Browne as a subject for literary biography – in an essay prefacing some of Browne's late works published in 1756 – long before he put together his compendious *Lives of the English Poets*. Though not alike in appearance or behaviour – Browne fastidious, Johnson famously a man of appetites – they had been at the same Oxford college, and shared at a century's distance a philosophy of life in which it wasn't Browne who was ahead of his time so much as Johnson who found himself out of tune with the Enlightenment, longing for days of certain religion and a human soul unchallenged by science.

Then there was the business of words. Browne must have caused him many a headache when Johnson was at work on the dictionary that would bring him lasting fame.

There had been dictionaries before. Thomas Blount's dictionary, published in 1656, was the best available in Browne's day. Blount's title – *Glossographia; or, a Dictionary Interpreting the Hard Words of Whatsoever Language, Now Used in Our English Tongue* – tells you all you need to know about what was happening to the language. It contained some 11,000 'hard' words, most of them added to the language during the preceding century, and was the largest dictionary of English at that time, until it was extensively plagiarized and enlarged two years later. (A more radical approach to the lexical chaos of the day was to start again with language altogether. In 1647, a Dutch-born London merchant, Francis Lodwick, published a manifesto for a utopian language that would permit people of different tongues to understand one another.)

Johnson's dictionary increased the number of words four-fold and improved the quality of the definitions with often pungent accuracy. Words came, as Blount had found already, from everywhere. Well travelled, multilingual and all curious, Browne was able to find enough raw material to make him one of the chief inventors of words in the seventeenth century. Words such as *electricity*, as well as *hallucination*, coined by Browne, had found their place in the language by Johnson's time and went into the dictionary. So did others now mostly obscure to us – the fabulous *retromingent*, for example, which means urinating rearwards. Other coinages – the superfluous *tollutation*, meaning simply ambling, the overly specific *axungious*, meaning lard-like – were rejected. Even the splendid *deuteroscopy*, meaning the business of taking a second look (always a Brownean urge), did not make it. Though Browne had a taste for Latinate car crashes – something later critics found a problem with Johnson too – his words were at least purposeful. As Johnson was forced to admit: 'in defence of his uncommon words and expressions, we must consider, that he had uncommon sentiments, and was not content to express in many words that idea for which any language could supply a single term'.

The compilers of the modern *Oxford English Dictionary* have computers to help them in their work, and are able to monitor the creation and usage of words. Browne ranks twenty-fifth among all sources responsible for providing first evidence of a word in English. He comes behind Shakespeare, Chaucer and King Alfred the Great, but well ahead of Spenser, Milton and Sir Francis Bacon. Scientific journals from all eras score highly; the *Philosophical Transactions of the Royal Society*, published continuously since 1665, turns out to be the second most fertile source of new words in the English language. The only individuals who outrank Browne among his contemporaries and near contemporaries are the handful of early lexicographers, Blount among them, and translators whose very business it was to pilot foreign words into English.

Science demanded names for things newly discovered or for the first time properly described – plants and animals, microorganisms visible through new microscopes, heavenly bodies visible through new telescopes. Bacon, the leading natural philosopher of the Elizabethan period, hoped that new words would define things with precision, a noun for each unique object in creation. Browne instinctively knew that words are slipperier than that. Science needs words that name but also words that describe. He favoured adjectives and adverbs, words that would do this job, but words also of polysemous possibility and ambiguity. For him, a good word was one that was more sayable, more poetic, more elaborately amusing, or more clearly bespeaking its classical origin as much as one that was blunt and clear.

Browne coined 784 new words and provided the first evidence for the true sense of another 1,616. The vast majority of them are found in the work of his that is most neglected by scholars of English literature, *Pseudodoxia Epidemica*. From his time in France, Italy and the Spanish Netherlands, Browne was well placed to make his contribution. The high jinks of his student days often shows through in these adoptions. He thought it worth importing *bouffage*, the French for a blowout or feast, and *saltimbanco*, a word heard in Italy that he clearly liked, used to describe a quack, literally a man who jumps up on a bench to make his sale.

Unlike Shakespeare, he seldom buds a new word from English roots, although he does come up with the delightful *swaggy* to describe the 'swaggy and prominent belly' of the beaver, and brings *stingy* out of Norfolk dialect into national usage. Most of Browne's neologisms come from Latin or Greek. Many are medical terms, and indeed Browne is the first to employ the word *medical*. He is responsible for our adoption of the Latin *incisor* to describe our cutting teeth. Terms such as *follicle* and *expectoration*, a word still used chiefly by doctors to mean coughing that produces phlegm, have been more thoroughly anglicized.

Admittedly, many of Browne's words are on the long side. Bored with the tedious phrase 'before the flood' in essays where he considers the veracity of biblical assertions about the significance of rainbows, the nature of the animals taken aboard the Ark and Methuselah's great age, he invents *antediluvian* to do the job. We still use it, though. He is guilty, too, of creating Latinisms where a more natural English alternative exists. Why invent *cecutiency* to mean near-blindness, out of the Latin *caecus* for blind, when purblindness exists already? Often, the answer lies in literary effect. In refuting the belief that moles are completely blind, he needed a balancing alliteration to make the sentence trip along that could not have been supplied by the obvious words: 'There is in them [moles] no Cecity, yet more then a Cecutiency.' In other words, they are not completely blind, but very nearly so, more than purblind.

It would not be fair to characterize such moments as mere verbal display. For Browne has in this passage not only already raised the topic of blindness or near-blindness in moles more plainly, but he also follows this abstruse sentence with the clearest possible amplification: 'they have sight enough to discern the light, though not perhaps to distinguish objects or colours; so they are not exactly blind, for light is one object of vision'. This oscillation between enthusiastic loquaciousness – his unfamiliar words almost always have a compensatory tongue-rolling sensuousness about them – and scientific lucidity is a chief identifying feature of Browne's unique style. Many of the words Browne devised in order to meet his exacting needs for description are with us still today, especially his new adverbial forms of words already in use as adjectives (*circumstantially, considerably, improbably, invariably, presumably, traditionally, horizontally* and *vertically*). Like Shakespeare and Milton, he also created many novel negatives by putting in- or un- in front of established words. They include *inactivity, inconsistent, indisputably* and *uncultivated*, though also *unridiculous* and *unquarrellable*, which over time have demonstrated their *unnecessity*.

A great many of Thomas Browne's neologisms are now even commoner words that we would not be without today: *append, aquiline, biped*, both *carnal* and *carnivorous, coexistence, compensate, equitable, exhaustion, ferocious, indigenous, insecurity, invigorate, locomotion, migrant* (as both noun and adjective), *misconception, prefix, pubescent, temperamental, ulterior, variegation* and *veterinarian*. He coined the terms *typographer* and *cryptography*. His need to describe geometrical arrangements caused him to invent *cylindrical* and *rhomboidal*. His discussion of the properties of magnets led him to coin the word *polarity*. *Electricity* sprang from his observations of the effects of static charges.

A word such as *deleterious* perfectly illustrates where Browne's inventions find their place. That it is a polysyllabic confection with a whiff of pedantry is not unusual for him. Nevertheless, deleterious has become a word we often see and use. Obviously, it means 'bad'. In fact, in many uses, bad would be a better word simply for being four syllables shorter. But we also know that its meaning is more nuanced than this, and it is generally used in this proper way that reflects its Greek root meaning noxious or hurtful, with the implication of working ill effects over a period of time. Browne used deleterious in relation to the action of poisons. As I write, it is chiefly used to describe the effects of domestic violence and environmental pollution and the side effects of drugs.

Denny Hilton, one of the editors of the *Oxford English Dictionary*, tells me: 'Browne is one of the most brilliant and prolific wordsmiths in the English language.' Hilton came across *Pseudodoxia Epidemica* by accident while at university, and was hooked by Browne's 'mix of scientific scrutiny and baroque style'. 'Most lexicographers have a soft spot for Browne,' he says, 'I think because of the quality as much as the quantity of his many coinages. It's not just neologistic showmanship – his words are complicated, minutely detailed, and lovingly created.'

The invention of new words continues today, of course, and the sources and processes involved are not dissimilar to those of Browne's time. The need to describe new scientific phenomena, as well as new technologies, is a driving force. Cross-cultural connections fertilize new words as they have always done, but at a greater rate owing to the speed of travel and communication. The words themselves may serve more vulgar needs, but they come about by the same processes that Browne used to create his neologisms: the collision of different Latin roots (*celebutante*, for example, or *edutainment*, a word that might have been invented to describe Browne's own prose), or the expedient addition of standard endings to convert one part of speech into another (*braggadocious*).

Words come into being when there is a need for them – when they describe new concepts to communicate to others – and they endure if those concepts continue to be of social importance. Browne's words inevitably tell us about the man. I cannot devote space to more examples here, but I have scattered a small lexicon of some of Browne's more successful words in footnotes at appropriate points throughout the remainder of this book.

It is of course not the new and unusual words but Browne's way with them that draws the praise of writers. They favour the candidly autobiographical *Religio Medici* and the rich humus of *Urne-Buriall*. For the most part, they ignore *Urne-Buriall*'s counterpart *The Garden of Cyrus*, which throws them off with its abrupt shifts between nature rhapsody, lists of plants, and odd ideas about their shape. *Pseudodoxia Epidemica* is also avoided because of its exhaustive length, its earnest mission, and because Browne is there less concerned with creating a literary effect.

So who joins Johnson in praising Browne? In his *Marginalia* Samuel Taylor Coleridge includes the transcription of a handwritten note he made in an edition of Browne's works: 'among my first favourites. Rich in various knowledge; exuberant in conceptions and conceits; contemplative, imaginative; often truly great and magnificent in his style and diction…he is a quiet and sublime *enthusiast*, with a strong tinge of the *fantast*; the humorist constantly mingling with, and flashing across the philosopher.' To Coleridge, Browne doesn't wander off his topic as other critics have been infuriated to find; he does the inverse of that, 'he metamorphoses all nature into it'.

In 1848, Herman Melville borrowed a copy of *Religio Medici* from his friend the publisher Evert Duyckinck. He decided that Browne was 'a crack'd Archangel' – a strange label, if presumably a flattering one. The context of the men's correspondence was a discussion of the American Transcendentalist authors, who were all 'cracked right across the brow' in Melville's view. He believed that his generation of writers owed a great debt to the fantastical imaginations of two centuries earlier. 'Lay it down that had not Sir Thomas Browne lived, Emerson would not have mystified.'

Melville was at work on *Moby-Dick* at this time, and was inspired by Browne's fidelity to nature as much as his fondness for 'mystification'. Some years after the first publication of *Pseudodoxia Epidemica* in 1646, a large sperm whale was stranded on the beach at Wells on the north Norfolk coast. Browne went to inspect the animal and was able to add a new chapter, 'Of Sperma-Ceti, and the Sperma-Ceti Whale', to the third edition in 1658. He describes the beast's anatomy and gives details of features sufficient to distinguish it from other whale species. He also takes samples of residues from the carcass, including the precious spermaceti, for experiment and further description of its distillation products.

Much of this material washes up again in Melville's long, scientifi-cally descriptive chapter 'Cetology', and elsewhere in *Moby-Dick*. But a truly Brownean thread is set running in a later chapter, 'Jonah Histori-cally Regarded'. Citing Nantucket whalers' supposed disbelief in the biblical truth of the story of Jonah and the whale, Melville applies his own scepticism through the character of an old whaler known by the name Sag-Harbor. Sag-Harbor doubts the story because he has seen illustrated Bibles that depict whales erroneously with two spouts as well as for other reasons drawn from his direct experience of whales and the sea. He is incredulous, too, that Jonah was swallowed some-where in the Mediterranean Sea and then regurgitated three days later at Nineveh, which would have required the whale to make an absurdly speedy passage round the Cape of Good Hope. But Melville does not allow Sag-Harbor's reason to prevail, and gives the last word to a priest who considers the whale's impossible journey 'a signal magnification of the general miracle'.

It is the antiquarian in Browne that enthrals Virginia Woolf. 'We are in the presence of sublime imagination; now rambling through one of the finest lumber rooms in the world – a chamber stuffed from floor to ceiling with ivory, old iron, broken pots, urns, unicorns' horns, and magic glasses full of emerald lights and blue mystery,' she writes in 1925 in *The Common Reader*. The rest of Browne hardly interests her at all, to judge by her review of a new *Works of Sir Thomas Browne* published a couple of years before this collection. She nods to one other work only, and that is of course *Religio Medici*. Even though Woolf showed far more interest in science than was generally considered healthy for a novelist, Browne's works of science do not merit a mention.

Woolf makes this surprising claim for Browne: 'His immense egotism has paved the way for all psychological novelists, autobiographers, confession-mongers, and dealers in the curious shades of our private life. He it was who first turned from the contacts of men with men to their lonely life within.' It is a curious remark not only because Browne is in many ways so unegotistical, but also because his 'life within' was surely less lonely than most. Besides it is not true. There is the important precedent of Montaigne, who, as Woolf herself says, has the advantage of a lucidity not yet found in English prose. She might have thought to mention also the visionary Margery Kempe of Bishop's Lynn (now King's Lynn) or the anchoress Julian of Norwich, both women writing autobiographically in the late medieval period. (Perhaps Norfolk breeds egotists.) Even so, Woolf does offer a needed counterweight to those who have skimmed Browne and found him melancholy. She sees his 'gusto' and love of life. 'In the midst of the solemnities of the Urn Burial we smile,' she says.

W.G. Sebald describes the reader's sensation precisely in his East Anglian meditation *The Rings of Saturn*: 'It is true that, because of the immense weight of the impediments he is carrying, Browne's writing can be held back by the force of gravitation, but when he does succeed in rising higher and higher through the circles of his spiralling prose, borne aloft like a glider on warm currents of air, even today the reader is overcome by a sense of levitation.' It is this abundant feeling of the light breaking through the heavy – levitation over gravitation, like the appearance of crepuscular rays of sunlight through dark clouds – that constantly rewards the reader.

More than once, reading through Browne's oeuvre, I have come away with a vision of Browne's personal levitation. He seems to have an aerial view at a time when aerial views were impossible. He feels the very orbit of the earth – or rather the constant slippage of the earth beneath the orbit of the sun, for he was not a convinced Copernican. It happens in a celebrated passage as he signs off at the end of *The Garden of Cyrus* and readies us for bed – or death: 'The Huntsmen are up in America, and they are already past their first sleep in Persia. But who can be drowsie at that howr which freed us from everlasting sleep? Or have slumbring thoughts at that time, when sleep it self must end, as some conjecture all shall awake again?'

Browne survives largely in quotes such as this. Modern readers may imagine that his writing is all like this, or that there is no argument to link together these rich passages. Is it that he is finally brought down, like his contemporary Cyrano de Bergerac, by his panache? Is it his sheer joy in language that makes us so suspicious of him today?

Edmund Gosse wrote a full biography of Browne on the tercentenary of his birth in 1905. It is workmanlike but unsympathetic, and betrays such a tin ear for the music of Browne's prose that Lytton Strachey rushed to Browne's defence. Gosse's work should perhaps be seen as a tentative approach to the confrontation with his preacher-naturalist father that would come with his famous autobiography, *Father and Son*, two years later. Gosse warms to his subject occasionally, not least when he appears to be a more sympathetic figure than his own father. Browne 'deprecated the frown of theology,' he writes with feeling. 'But he knew by experience that people love to preserve their mistakes, and are often heartily vexed to be set right.' That 'by experience' is a key to Browne, the practising physician, accustomed to reasoning with patients at the bedside, and to knowing when further reasoning will do no good. Today I feel compelled to add that he would have deprecated also the frown of the overzealous advocate of science.

The Argentinian writer Jorge Luis Borges set out on his career by doing his 'best to be Sir Thomas Browne'. Browne makes a brief appearance at the very end of Borges's short story 'Tlön, Uqbar, Orbis Tertius', which centres on the discovery of one volume (Hlaer–Jangr) of a multi-volume encyclopedia that seems to be the key to a vanished civilization, Tlön. It transpires that the civilization itself is a fiction concocted by a secret society in the early seventeenth century – a later member of the society, Borges tells us, was the Irish philosopher George Berkeley, whose theory of immaterialism denied the existence of physical matter. There are shades of *Urne-Buriall* here and also of a playful late work of Browne's, *Musaeum Clausum*, a catalogue of objects that he thought should exist, but which definitely didn't. After the hoax has been revealed, the narrator of Borges's story is found in the last sentence endlessly revising his translation of *Urne-Buriall*, working his passage back to the seventeenth century. 'The world will be Tlön,' he announces.

I can find no scholarship explicitly linking Vladimir Nabokov to Browne, but when I see the first sentence of his autobiography *Speak, Memory* I feel I am reading a Browne updated for the atheistic present: 'The cradle rocks above an abyss, and common sense tells us that our existence is but a brief crack of light between two eternities of darkness.'

Browne's most renowned literary champion today is the Spanish novelist Javier Marías. Marías has also confessed to refining his style by translating various English classics, including *Tristram Shandy* and the works of Robert Louis Stevenson, Thomas Hardy and W. H. Auden. In a delicious Borgesian twist, Marías's translations of Browne are now available under the imprint 'Reino de Redonda' since Marías is the reigning King of Redonda. It seems as if it must be a fictional title, but Redonda actually exists. Indeed, I have seen it while standing on the Caribbean island of Nevis, a green-lidded chunk of volcanic rock lying a few miles across the glittering sea. The monarchy stretches back to 1880 when the Montserrat-born M. P. Shiel, an Edwardian writer of fantasies, staged an imaginative coup and first claimed the crown. Under King Xavier, as Marías has styled himself, this tropical Rockall has been transformed into a Tlön-like refuge of literary civilization, with the appointment as peers of the realm of A. S. Byatt, Umberto Eco, Philip Pullman and others. The king's translation of Browne is dedicated to Sebald, 'Duke of *Vertigo* and invisible friend, who wrote extraordinary pages on Sir Thomas Browne and met death unwished on a road in Norfolk, not far from the buried and unearthed urns.'

Perhaps Marías himself can tell me why Browne so appeals to some writers. I write to him – my first royal correspondence – and am thrilled a few days later to receive a detailed reply to my questions, personally typewritten, then electronically scanned and forwarded to me by his assistant. Marías discovered Browne when studying English literature in Spain. Finding himself agreeably challenged by the prose, he translated *Religio Medici*, *Urne-Buriall* and a note on dreams for a Madrid publisher of classics, although he nearly abandoned the project. 'I am happy I did not, of course, and certainly I know his style has had an influence in some of my writing. As it were, I feel capable of "introducing" in my own writing what might be called "the Browne pitch": a certain gravity, a certain nobility of style, as well as a certain serenity.' Marías was gratified by sales of his translations, but gives the greater credit to Sebald. 'The funny thing is that some Spanish writers "discovered" Browne with Sebald, not knowing they had a much older translation of some of his works into Spanish. Perhaps, thanks to Sebald (with whom I exchanged a few letters before his death), Browne came to be known a little more here.' Marías's letter ends with a sentiment that I know to be true: 'he has stayed with me during all these years, and I think he shall stay forever'.

Death looms large in the American playwright Tony Kushner's 'epic farce' *Hydriotaphia*, in which the action takes place on Browne's last day on earth. 'Hydriotaphia' is Browne's Hellenic synonym invented as an alternative title for *Urne-Buriall*. Though I have not seen a production and must reach my judgement off the page, the play presents a Browne I scarcely recognize. It is at least a speculation about mortality, like Browne's original. But Kushner has conflated death with money in a very unBrownean – though very twentieth-century Brechtian – way, by making Browne the magnate of a local stone quarry (a preposterous idea in Norfolk where the only stone to be extracted from the ground is flint).

Reviews of the few productions tend to the view that Kushner has over-reached himself. Any drama that includes the line spoken by Browne, 'You who must live through this, I pity you', is asking for a rough ride.

I am not sure how I feel about following this company. I love *Moby-Dick* and have read some Virginia Woolf, respectfully admiring her stylistic innovation. I have wrestled with a few of the teasing, complex tales of Borges. But the fact is these are mostly not my favourite authors, and they are a heterogeneous bunch.* But we share our fandom, and fans are family who can cross boundaries of time and taste. Perhaps it is a hint that I should pick up some Emerson.

However, I have just cause to shoulder my way in among these writers. I have hinted that they have largely ignored the bulk of Browne's output, and the part that was most successful in his lifetime, the writing about what was not yet called science. This is a forgivable omission on the part of those whose first (or second) interest is not science, but it does a disservice to Browne.

Unfortunately, Browne is just as missing from the literature of science. I search almost in vain for scientists and science writers who feel the need to invoke his name for any reason. I cannot find him in the works of Carl Sagan, who debunked the vulgar errors of his own age in *The Demon-Haunted World*, while Richard Dawkins is predictably curt on Browne's apparent love of mystery. I am delighted when I find that Stephen Jay Gould praises him in *The Mismeasure of Man*, his masterly condemnation of the pseudoscience that aims to sort people by racial and other types. He does so not only because Browne is 'almost maximally philo-Semitic by the standards of his century', but because he finds his writing 'strangely fascinating'. Most of all, though, Gould

---

* Seeing the closing words of *Urne-Buriall*, recommending modesty in death, and that any of us should be 'as content with six foot as the Moles of Adrianus' (that is, the grandiose tomb of the Emperor Hadrian in Rome, now crowned by the Castel Sant'Angelo), I became excited by the idea that even the late Sue Townsend was a fan, and had been inspired to name her eponymous teenage diarist Adrian Mole after reading Browne, until I found that her first thought had been to call him Nigel, and the fancy withered.

wishes to draw our attention to the way in which Thomas Browne is able to marshal a rational argument in *Pseudodoxia Epidemica*, which unexpectedly turns up 'a layer of modern relevance'.

You have to go back another generation or two to find more of Browne's scientific champions. Charles Mackay mentions him in a detailed scrutiny of the 1662 Bury witch trial in his famous work *Extraordinary Popular Delusions and the Madness of Crowds* of 1841, but only reports the 'evidence' he gave there; it would have been interesting to hear his opinion of Browne's testimony. William Ramsay, the chemist who added five new elements, the noble gases, to the periodic table, placed an epigraph from *Religio Medici* at the top of the paper summarizing his achievements: '*Natura nihil agit frustra*, is the only indisputed Axiome in Philosophy. There are no Grotesques in Nature; not anything framed to fill up the empty Canons, and unnecessary Spaces.' The Canadian physician Sir William Osler, one of the founders of the famous Johns Hopkins Hospital in Baltimore, and the physician who introduced bedside patient experience into the curriculum for medical students, regarded Browne as a lifelong role model. Toasting the unveiling of Browne's statue in Norwich in 1905, he identified three lessons from his life, the most astute of these being his overseas education, which led to his being 'denationalized as far as his intellect and his human sympathies were concerned'. D'Arcy Thompson, the classicist, mathematician and zoologist, author of the brilliant and erudite *On Growth and Form*, refers his readers to Browne's 'quaint and beautiful' *The Garden of Cyrus* during the course of a detailed discussion of the symmetries observed in soap bubbles and honeycombs. He is able to explain mathematically why, as Browne noted, the leaves of some plants, such as hazel, grow in an unequal manner. Joseph Needham, the renowned author of the multi-volume *Science and Civilisation in China*, who began his career as a biochemist, regarded Browne as an unsung pioneer of chemical embryology, the science that aims to identify the stimuli that cause cells to differentiate as they develop into adult organisms.

There may be more such votaries I have not discovered, but the pattern emerges already. Browne is admired most by those who, like him, are great in places they have chosen for themselves on the fringes and in the interstices between conventional disciplines.

*

Chronicling a new form of carbon in 1992 opened a window for me to a fresh view of science, one of recurrent motifs and patterns that are present in nature at all times and at all scales, and that reveal themselves only when we have the equipment or the preparedness to look in the right direction.

A little later, I moved to Norfolk, and found Browne waiting for me. I felt that if I could understand Browne more deeply – Browne who had left London and Oxford and the best universities on the continent to settle in Norwich – it might help me make sense of my own new life in the remote and strange county of Norfolk. Of course, he had his medical profession – his writing was always done on the side. But did he not feel his disconnection, his remoteness from the hub of the action? His seclusion seems not to have bothered him at all. It is clear that he preferred to organize his thoughts in his own way rather than in the way dictated by the *Philosophical Transactions of the Royal Society*. The scientific paper was never going to be his preferred literary form while there was the opportunity of a glorious discursive essay. And if the price he paid for that was a few minor discoveries not made, a few others not properly attributed to him, the odd professional friendship not formed, and being a little out of date here and there, then so be it.

In Norfolk, I hatched an idea to put on an exhibition to commemorate the quatercentenary of his birth in 2005. Although by then I knew a little about him, it seemed that the most famous cultural figure ever to have come out of Norwich was unknown to most of its citizens. With no obvious single venue, I conceived of five little exhibitions scattered around the city, each one in a location appropriate to one of Browne's thematic preoccupations and to one of his books. Browne's scientific debunking of 'vulgar errors' was to be celebrated at a 'hands on' children's science centre, his medical career at the Norfolk and Norwich Hospital, his observations of pattern and form in plant growth at the John Innes Centre, a world-renowned horticultural research institute. The cathedral would address his still pertinent views on religion expressed in his youthful *Religio Medici* and the later *Christian Morals*. Best of all, I had managed to interest the Sainsbury Centre for Visual Arts, where I thought a display of burial urns would resonate perfectly with their superb collection of modern pottery. The five locations would make a quincunx on any map of Norwich. But my plan went nowhere. Later I learnt that the city had chosen to mark the anniversary by commissioning a large public sculpture, which was installed some years late next to the statue erected on the previous centenary. Who Browne really was and what he stood for, what he wrote and the way he wrote, would have to be explained in other ways, or not at all.

And so I dare to follow these illustrious earlier champions of Browne because, like them, I have become enchanted by his prose, but also because there is a job to do. Browne's genuine contribution to science is under-appreciated. Furthermore, his way of writing for the scientifically ignorant, always tolerant and forgiving, humorous and elegant, is a model for today. It offers an urgently needed alternative to the arrogant and impatient tone of many communicators of science. This tension is especially evident where science impinges on domains, such as religion and politics, where subjective opinions may be valued as much as the 'objective' ones of science, and where the debate has sometimes grown excessively shrill. Here Browne can bring wisdom to bear.

I understand that it is not enough for me to point out a few passages of his writing and ask how they apply today. I must show how a modern-day Thomas Browne would approach these problems. How would he tackle the 'vulgar errors' of today? What, indeed, are these errors? We might imagine we are so enlightened that we no longer labour under such delusions. But in some ways, the situation may actually be worse than in Browne's day. His ostensible readers had some justification for holding to their superstitious beliefs because they had little or no education, and certainly none in natural philosophy. (I say 'ostensible' because

Pseudodoxia Epidemica was of course read chiefly by Browne's clever peers, just as today's science polemicists preach largely to the converted.) Today's 'vulgar errors' are perpetrated by people who ought to know better, people who have acquired at least the rudiments of science at school but who nevertheless visit chiropractors, pursue homoeopathic remedies, refuse their children the MMR vaccine, believe that crystals have special powers, and deny the likelihood of climate change. What would he say to them? Would he be as harsh as today's self-appointed megaphones for science? And what would he have to say about science and religion, the two forces that he sought to reconcile in *Religio Medici*? Would he perhaps, like many scientists, be an atheist today? Or does his settlement leave room for both rationalism and faith? And if it does, would he be able to win over both the Archbishop of Canterbury and Richard Dawkins?

If this is not to be a more or less chronological biography – and the scarcity of known facts about Thomas Browne throughout his life means that it cannot be – then it is hard to avoid chapters based on his varied published works. However, as these will be unfamiliar to many readers, I have not taken this path. Instead, following brief sketches of his life and professional milieu, each chapter takes as its theme an idea that was important to Browne, and that I believe is also important to us now. In this way, I range from medicine, medical care and human longevity to natural history, science and human culture. My examination of both scientific and unscientific ways of looking at the world leads me, a one-time scientist, naturally enough to consider the tolerance we show, or do not, towards people who do not think like us. This structural decision allows me to slip more freely between the seventeenth and the twenty-first centuries in order to show how Browne's philosophy bears on our lives and beliefs today. I find that he brings fresh insight into contemporary debate, not only where we might expect it, such as on the relation between science and religion, but also where we might not, such as in relation to our mental health and happiness and the culture of consumerism in which we are so thoroughly immersed.

I must add one more author to my list of Browne's literary admirers. In a short story, E. M. Forster makes Thomas Browne the driver of 'The Celestial Omnibus', in which a suburban boy boards the bus for a day trip to heaven. The driver introduces himself – 'His face was a surprise, so kind it was and modest' – accepts no fare, and the boy finds himself rising heavenwards through thunderclouds, pulled by two horses which have feasted on 'clovers of Latinity'. He might not stick to the advertised route or arrive punctually at his destination, but he can be relied upon to get us to the right place. I can think of nobody better to lead us on such a journey.

I

Biography

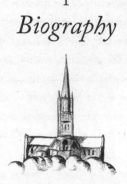

'Embryon philosopher'

Urne-Buriall

THOMAS BROWNE DIED on 19 October 1682, seventy-seven years to
the day from his birth in 1605. 'Sr Tho: Browne is dead, & as hee
lived in an eaven temper without deep concerne with how the world
went, & was therein in very happy so hee dyed like a wise old philosopher,' wrote Thomas Townshend to Horatio, Lord Townshend, of
Raynham Hall with the news.

The curious fact of dying on the anniversary of one's birth was something that Browne had characteristically taken the time to investigate. At
some time during the 1650s, it seems, he wrote an essay that has become
known as 'A Letter to a Friend'. Addressed to an unknown recipient, it
is headed in full 'to a friend, upon occasion of the death of his intimate
friend'. In it Browne strives to offer some comfort to his bereaved correspondent. But it is a raw kind of comfort he brings, for along with the
conventional platitudes he does not shun the facts of death. His obsequies rise up in poetic flights while his medical realism continually brings
us back down to the mortician's slab, occasionally in the same sentence.

He recollects a few of the unpleasant deaths to which he has been
witness as a physician, and which he has read about in ancient accounts.

The alarming variety of human ends then tempts him to a comparison with beginnings: 'With what strife and pains we came into the World we know not; but 'tis commonly no easie matter to get out of it.' Noting that the lost friend died 'when the Moon was in motion from the Meridian' – that is to say rising in the sky, a time when disproportionate numbers of people once were thought to die – he moves from speculations about the favoured hour for the births and deaths of animals and men, and the high prevalence of infants dying on their natal day, to more noteworthy coincidences. The Holy Roman Emperor Charles V was supposedly crowned on his birthday, for example.

But the greatest synchrony that can shape a human life on earth is surely that the lifespan should mesh perfectly with the planet's orbit around the sun. As Browne puts it: 'But in Persons who out-live many Years, and when there are no less than three hundred and sixty-five days to determine their Lives in every Year; that the first day should make the last, that the Tail of the Snake should return into its Mouth precisely at that time, and they should wind up on the day of their Nativity, is indeed a remarkable Coincidence.'

Is it, though? Browne clearly savours the idea of a person's dying on their birthday for its own sake. He is alive to the symmetry it seems to bring to a life. If 'our little life / Is rounded with a sleep', as Prospero says in *The Tempest*, what more perfect circularity could there be than this? Surely, none. But is it actually a remarkable coincidence that it should happen?

We would naturally expect that 1 in 365 of us (or 4 in 1461, to allow for leap years) dies on this special day, or for that matter on Christmas Day or any given day of the year. Browne does not suggest that dying on this day is significant or **anomalous**; it is merely 'remarkable'. He notes the neatness of the coincidence, but does not imply that more people

❧❧❧❧❧❧❧❧❧❧ ❧ ❧ ❧❧❧❧❧❧❧❧❧❧

anomalous (PE, 1646): Browne delighted in the anomalous and the odd (anomalous is derived from the Greek for un-even). The sighting of a rare species, the digging up of a puzzling antiquity, the patient with an unusual condition is always worthy of proper die on this day than simple arithmetic would lead us to expect, nor that fewer do so. Yet the coincidence would only be truly remarkable if a *disproportionate* number of people die on their birthday, that is to say if either rather more or rather less than 1 person in every 365 achieves this peculiar feat. As we shall see, this is a matter that modern-day statisticians have struggled to address.

You would think Browne was born with the knighthood. The 'Sir' prefaces his name on all his books. Biographical accounts refer to him as Sir Thomas Browne on his continental journeys, at Oxford, even as a schoolboy at Winchester. But he was not 'Sir' then. His family had no hereditary baronetcy.

In fact, the honour came late in life and was conferred, like many a Stuart knighthood, more or less on a whim. In September 1671, Charles II visited Norwich, as well as the port of Yarmouth, which was making important preparations for war against the Dutch. It seems that it was a chance meeting, and the king's need to distribute honours according to custom, that led to the award. Browne had no particular business with the king other than perhaps providing a few medical certificates for tuberculous cases to be put forward to be touched for the king's evil. So it was that Browne acquired a title that better-remembered men of science and letters – William Harvey, Robert Hooke, John Donne, John Milton – never did.

The unusually adhesive title is not only a happy gesture of deference to an admirable man but is also, as I realize when I set a Google Alert, a necessary filter. There are simply too many Thomas Brownes. The knighthood is a fitting badge of his uniqueness. (As E. M. Forster wrote, 'it does serve to distinguish one Jack from his fellow'.) However, it is not necessary to keep making that distinction here, and I shall for

observation and recording. Underlying description is the urge towards classification, the triumphant placing of the anomalous within man's system of nature that would become the driving impulse of early modern science.

the most part return him to the common ranks.

Thomas Browne was born in London, in the parish of St Michael, Cheapside. His father, Thomas, was a successful silk merchant who died when his son was eight years old. His mother, Anne, remarried Sir Thomas Dutton, whose social position, together with money which had been left in his father's will for the upbringing of his three sisters as well as young Thomas, secured Browne the best education of the day.

At the age of eleven, he obtained a scholarship to Winchester College, where he remained until he was eighteen. He entered Broadgates Hall in Oxford in 1623. Shortly afterwards, it was renamed as Pembroke College, and he participated in a ceremony to mark the occasion, improbably (being only in his second undergraduate year) giving a Latin oration which already incorporates characteristic Brownean themes of ruination and rebirth, referring to 'this Phoenix of Pembroke uproused from the ruins of this very ancient hall'. His tutor was Thomas Lushington, a thinking preacher who ran into trouble with the university authorities over his sermons for advocating peace when many wanted war with Spain and for seeming to 'deal lightly with the sacred mystery of the Resurrection'.

The extended 'memo to self' that is *Religio Medici* contains some clues to Browne's character as a young man. He is 'bashfull' and diligent: 'I was bred in the way of study.' His conversation, he admits, can be 'austere, my behaviour full of rigour, sometimes not without morosity'. Although his university education is in the classical arts – logic, rhetoric, meta-physics and moral philosophy – he has been interested from an early age in science and medicine, collecting herbs around Cheapside during his holidays from school. He pretends laziness, he confesses minor heresies, he has committed sins, he says, but only the sins everyone commits. He has escaped the sin of pride, he tells us, moments before telling us that he can understand six languages as well as 'the *Jargon* and *Patois* of severall Provinces'. He takes pride, too, in his physique and good health as a young man, but is already mindful of death, finding himself 'as wholesome a morsell for the wormes as any'. But he has a robust constitution and is aware that he is in the prime of life – or rather, because he is given to indirectness, he is aware he is at that age when men typically feel that they are in the prime of life.

He believes he is easy-going: 'I am of a constitution so generall, that it consorts, and sympathizeth with all things; I have no antipathy, or rather Idio-syncrasie, in dyet, humour, ayre, any thing.' And he believes he is old before his time because he has the dreamlike sensation of being a spectator at life's feast, a feeling he knows he should resist. He will prosper as a physician, but he finds that he is more charitable when he himself is poor. He is baffled and greatly affected by the power of friendship, noting down remarks that echo Montaigne's on the subject, and he hints at one close friendship in particular. In moments of self-pity, with his father dead and his mother remarried, he denies it but desperately feels the want of close bonds. 'I doe not find in my selfe such a necessary and indissoluble Sympathy to all those of my bloud.' It would be good to have a family.

Many of the qualities that give Browne his unique voice, including his facility with languages, come with his subsequent medical training on the continent. His first trip abroad, though, was a tour of Ireland with his stepfather, who owned estates there. Little information survives about this journey, but he did notice that there were spiders, which enabled him to put down an English myth that there weren't. This trivial episode displays the traits that Browne was to make his own: the commitment to seeing with his own eyes, and the mental alertness to transfer what is accepted in one place and use it to counter superstition in another.

Medicine gives him the opportunity to complete his studies in the best European universities, Montpellier, Padua, and Leiden, where at last he receives his doctoral degree. He enjoys debating with his teachers. He takes on 'a Doctor of Physick in Italy, who could not perfectly believe the immortality of the soule' because it was not to be found in Galen, the Roman physician whose ideas still dominated medicine. In France, he finds a theologian troubled on the same point by lines of Seneca, who famously wrote that there is nothing after death, and death itself is nothing. Browne falls easily into conversation with any divine who will give him the time of day, and it is obvious even in his own rendition of these encounters that they often weary of his puppyish mind games. In his earnest youth, it seems Browne may have been a bit of a bore defending his Christian faith against new philosophies. But he listens and learns as much as he talks and brings back what he has learnt.

Then in his late twenties Browne makes an abrupt retreat. He returns to England and settles in Shibden Dale near Halifax in Yorkshire. There are good reasons for this – he cannot yet practise medicine in places such as Oxford or London before his Dutch doctorate has been formally recognized.

But moving to Shibden Dale seems to be taking extreme measures. He found a position at Shibden Hall. It is not an easy place to locate. Examining the maps, I find there is a Shibden Hall, which is a fifteenth-century estate open to the public as a museum and gallery. But this is not the place. It was once known as Lower Shibden Hall to distinguish it from Upper Shibden Hall, which then squatted on an exposed hillside a mile or so further up the dale. And this is where Browne supposedly lived and worked. The house on the site today has fallen into decay, but is Georgian in any case. There is no trace of the

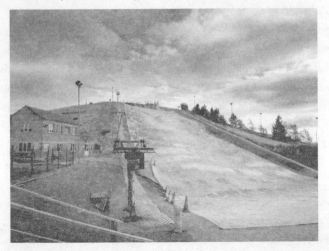

building Browne would have known. The chief landmark is an abandoned dry ski slope on the hilltop that seems to stand for lost hope.

A doctor will find patients deserving of medical attention wherever he goes, of course. He would be needed here. But he would be needed anywhere. Why here? What led Browne to this bleak spot? Probably some family connection or Oxford contact with the hall. But there must be something more. Browne has the training to become one of the great scientists* of the period. All he needs is to surround himself with like minds. But he does not do this. Something about the life does not suit him. He finds instead a place for introspection ideal for working up the magnificent, solipsistic masterpiece that will be *Religio Medici*, 'penned in such a place and with such disadvantage, that…I had not the assistance of any good booke'.† Here he synthesizes all he believes and all he has learnt. Not everything fits. Incompatible views crash up against each other. No matter. Get it down anyway.

In 1637, after the required fourteen years had elapsed following his matriculation, Oxford University incorporated his Leiden doctoral degree. He was now free to practise where he chose. He chose Norwich. Again, it is not clear why. Again, it seems likely that he was urged by contacts and friends, including his Oxford tutor, Lushington. Norwich was prosperous and cosmopolitan. It was a step towards the centre, the only one he would take. He took premises on the street then and now called Tombland (a Viking inheritance, it means 'open place' and has nothing to do with tombs). Here, just outside the cathedral walls, he began to attend to the people of Norfolk as he would for the remaining forty-five years of his life.

---

* I use the terms science, scientific and the professional label of scientist to apply to Browne, recognizing that they are strictly anachronistic – the words will not be coined or used in the senses that we use them today for a century or more – because Browne is nevertheless so obviously a kind of scientist.
† This episode in Browne's life is only asserted in recent scholarship, and evidence of his presence in Shibden is not wholly reliable. One source is a doctor and debtor often in Halifax jail who was five years old during the time of Browne's sojourn. Another is a former curate of the parish. Both seem keener to claim that *Religio Medici* sprang from their soil than on accurate recollection of its author.

'I never yet cast a true affection on a Woman,' Browne writes, aged thirty, although he implies some familiarity with the sexual act, for he wishes that 'we might procreate like trees, without conjunction, or that there were any way to perpetuate the world without this trivial and vulgar way of coition; It is the foolishest act a wise man commits in all his life.' When he marries Dorothy Mileham in 1641, perhaps he finds it is also the means to our closest communication with another human soul. In any event, he is reconciled to the idea soon enough. Their first child, Edward, is born in 1644. In the first edition of *Pseudodoxia Epidemica* published in 1646, he makes clear he would not be without the consolations of married life, writing with pity of the predicament of the 'churchman…doomed to a life of celibacy by the **asceticism** which had corrupted the simplicity of Christianity'. Dorothy will bear him eleven children.

He regards women conventionally as the weaker sex. To the idea that God created woman as a helpmeet for man, he reckons the only help she really offers is 'unto generation; for as for any other help, it had been fitter to have made another man'. But this is disingenuous. He happily acknowledges and cites the work of learned women in his writing, and is open to the idea of female scholarship. In Italy, he will have been aware of a tradition of women appointed to chairs in physic at some of the universities.

Only five of their eleven children outlived Thomas and Dorothy. They are unlucky even by the standards of an age when a quarter were expected to die young, and more when the plague comes. The eldest child, Edward, and four sisters, Anne, Elizabeth, Mary and Frances, survived Sir Thomas.

❧❧❧❧❧❧❧❧❧❧❧ ❧ ❧ ❧❧❧❧❧❧❧❧❧❧

ascetic and **asceticism** (PE, 1646): These words occur in a surprising passage on the rights of women: 'This ascetic rule, which held that a saint was disgraced by the very society which his mild Master sought and loved, added the finishing stroke to woman's degradation.' I think we can be sure that Browne identified more with the saint than with the Master here. He was in many ways a typical man of his age, but not in his experience of its sensual aspect. He did not seek excess – of food, drink or sex. He would not have shared the king's love of fart jokes.

Five more children born between 1649 and 1656 died in infancy or early childhood. Young Tom, the second born, joined the navy and was lost a few years later, scarcely into his twenties, in unknown circumstances. It is just as well that Browne does not consider, as some people do, that having children is a path to immortality. Edward Browne's only son, another Thomas, died in 1711, just three years after his father. The Browne line was extinct within thirty years of Sir Thomas's death.

What did parents feel about the loss of a child when so many were lost? Was the grief less overwhelming? Are family sorrows a reason for Thomas's maudlin disquisitions on burial urns, the first of these published in 1658, shortly after the deaths of twin sons at the ages of just two months and fourteen months? Does melancholy need a reason? And can it even find a place today, squeezed in somewhere between society's need for us to keep smiling and a grief industry hovering by ready to tell us how to suffer?

The Brownes were a close and loving family. Paternal letters begin 'Dear Sonne' or sometimes 'D. S.' and typically conclude 'YLF' – 'your loving father'. They offer the usual wishes for good health, observations on medical matters, advice on places to see and to avoid, notes on shared enthusiasms and local news. 'The Epitome of Anatomie in English is come to Norwich,' Sir Thomas writes to Edward, who will become a physician like his father, and eventually president of the College of Physicians, and will count Charles II among his patients. But the lecture, he observes with breezy professionalism, is priced at sixpence '& will sell the slower'. Occasionally, there is a domestic postscript in the less polished hand of Dorothy, barely scraping the paper, reiterating her husband's good wishes and perhaps requesting some particular cloth from London.

Although the Brownes brought their family into the world during one of the most turbulent periods in English history – the Civil War, the Commonwealth and the Restoration – his references to these events are rare, and lead him into uncharacteristic grandiose comparisons. In the dedication of *Religio Medici*, which Browne has been driven to publish in 1643 because others have distributed unauthorized editions, Browne likens his difficulties with the fourth estate to those lately experienced by the other estates of the nation, 'the name of his Majesty defamed, the honour of Parliament depraved'. He refers to dangers escaped and turns of luck in his early years, presumably when he was on his travels. He does not tell us what these accidents were, but draws a portentous parallel between his moments of good fortune and that moment of national good fortune when the Gunpowder Plot was uncovered in the year of his birth. It is clear enough that Browne did not wish to see a return to Catholicism or the crown and parliament challenged or overthrown.

He understands – and fears – the power of the written word. 'I had rather stand in the shock of a Basilisco than in the fury of a Mercilesse Pen', he writes in *Religio Medici*. For he has had the unpleasant sensation of finding this very work published without his permission. That scholars' tongues are 'sharper than Actius his razor' he will feel directly several more times in his life, and notably when a rival physician, one Alexander Ross, pursues Browne with angry rebuttals of his work, publishing *Medicus Medicatus* ('A Doctor Doctored') in response to *Religio Medici*, and later, in answer to *Pseudodoxia Epidemica*, a lengthy diatribe called *Arcana Microcosmi* in which for good measure he takes on landmark works by Francis Bacon and William Harvey as well.

Standing on Mousehold Heath, the hillock of untamed land from which Robert Kett launched a rebellion, with the morning sun on your back, it is still easy to make out the Norwich Browne would have known. The vista closely matches early maps of the city with their combined plan and perspective views. Held in a tight bend of the River Wensum, the city spreads between its cubic Norman castle and, lying closer to, the bodkin spire of the cathedral, both executed in a foreign stone. Humbler buildings have grey flint walls and are roofed with thick clay tiles, materials which, taken together, serve to distinguish Norwich from other English cities. Many streets bear the Danish suffix -*gate* – Pottergate, Colegate, Fishergate; squares are called plains after the Dutch *plein*.

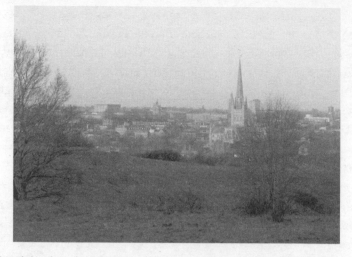

Dutch brickwork and stepped or shaped gables are the fashion in architecture; wavy pantiles, now ubiquitous, are just coming in. Even the land around the city is being transformed, with ditches dug and sluices put in under supervision of Dutch water engineers. The city walls – mostly still standing today, though little noticed – are ambitious in their circumference, enclosing an area larger than the city of London, an area too great to settle densely, so that by the seventeenth century Norwich is, according to the historian Thomas Fuller, 'either a City in an Orchard, or an Orchard in a City, so equally are Houses and Trees blended in it'.

Now, let us go down the hill, and across Bishop Bridge into the busy streets. The name of Norwich means a 'northern trading place'. In the seventeenth century it is England's second city, a thriving cosmopolis. The population is around 20,000 – and held constant throughout the century by periodic outbreaks of plague and other diseases which cancel the effect of migration from the countryside. With the river providing a still navigable link to the sea, there are numbers of Dutch and Flemish, Huguenot French and Walloons as well as Norwegians, Danes, Russians and Germans. For some of these, the city is a place of refuge and it prides itself on finding ways to assimilate what it calls its 'strangers'.

There is no court at Norwich and it is not an intellectual centre; its life is commerce. Men come to buy and sell. The Hanseatic League, which shaped trade in northern Europe during the medieval and early modern period, grew out of an alliance of German city states. The league's lifeblood was never nations or territories but the seaways linking trading partners across the North Sea and the Baltic. The league expanded rapidly to include ports from Novgorod in the east to Boston, Lincolnshire, in the west, and Bergen in the north to Cologne in the south. Yarmouth and King's Lynn became trading posts early on, even before London, and Norwich felt the benefit.

Norfolk has grown by exporting wool, although this lucrative trade has declined by the seventeenth century. In its place go new and fancy fabrics. In come timber and iron from Scandinavia and Saxony. This trade makes Norwich a greater commercial centre than Bristol until the advent of the Atlantic trade and greater than Birmingham or Manchester until the Industrial Revolution. The citizens have rare skills and are able to add value to the goods that pass through. Weavers and dyers produce constant innovations in fabrics – 'stuffs'. Bright colours are part of the appeal. There is still a street called St John Maddermarket, after the crimson dye extracted from the madder plant. Some fabrics are hot-pressed to give them a glossy sheen, another local speciality. Printers produce books, first in Dutch, later in English. There are moneylenders, street-sellers, painters, goldsmiths, clockmakers. Apothecaries are found in the lanes leading off the Market Place. The city is prosperous. It supports its own money market, a summer assizes and a winter theatre season. The city authorities are efficient and decent. It is a comparatively literate place, the first in England to open a civic library, in 1608.

In 1650, with his family growing, Thomas Browne is amid all this bustle. He has no scholarly retreat; his house is yards from the Market Place and the coaching inns. It is the market church of St Peter Mancroft where he worships. He can hear the street cries and the church bells as well as the gulls that scream over the city.

What still thrives of this Norwich? And what signs are there of the rest? The obvious clue to its historic prosperity and its multitudes then is not the Guildhall or the cathedral but the many churches. In 1724, Daniel Defoe counted thirty-two parishes within the city walls. A citizen of Norwich would have been hard put to walk more than a furlong to go to worship. Most of the churches still stand, some now deconsecrated and put to other uses – one is a concert hall, another a puppet theatre. One, Browne might have been interested to see, became the science discovery centre where I wanted to hold my exhibition, until forced to close for repair work on the tower. It is now vacant and to let. Another church provides a home for stalls selling bric-a-brac and collectibles. I notice second-hand copies of W. G. Sebald's *The Rings of Saturn* and Christopher Hitchens's *God is Not Great* sharing one table.

Norwich is still comparatively literate. It has resisted a national wave of library closures, and has recently been selected as a world City of Literature by UNESCO. It is still a trading place, too, not so visibly concerned with import and export now, but conspicuously dedicated to shopping. It has a vibrant cultural life but no real cultural centre. The focus is provided, as it long has been, by the vast marketplace, which is surrounded by malls and pedestrianized shopping streets. These thoroughfares are thronged during the day, but fall eerily quiet as soon as the shops shut. If you happen to glance above the display windows, you see that the city has buildings of every period from the medieval to the modern. There is very little poor architecture and the result makes a pleasing eclectic mix.

The population is actually less mixed than it was in the seventeenth century. In 2011 just over one in seven citizens of Norwich identified themselves, in that peculiar way demanded by the national census, as belonging to an ethnicity or national identity other than 'White: English/Welsh/Scottish/Northern Irish/British'. There is a smattering of other ethnicities, but the largest single remainder group is the 5.4 per cent who are 'White Other', perhaps the kind of 'strangers' who came to be tolerated in the seventeenth century. I spot a new Lithuanian restaurant. The Hanseatic League has been revived by Ryanair and EasyJet.

Outside the doors of the Primark on Gentleman's Walk, where Browne's property once extended, a man with wild greasy hair is having a hard time making giant soap bubbles, cursing his efforts in a Balkan tongue. A woman with a floral headband sets up a microphone and announces quietly 'I'm going to Wichita'. A man bawls in an African language into his mobile phone, making animated gesticulations as he does so, and bursting into English for occasional emphasis.

On Hay Hill, opposite the site of Browne's house and next to the church in which he worshipped, is the contemporary sculpture placed by the city to mark the four hundredth anniversary of Browne's birth. The French artists, Anne and Patrick Poirier, have carved a variety of

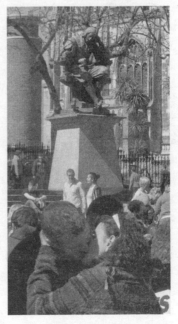

stones, many designed to be sat on and grouped so as to form an outdoor room. The 1905 bronze statue of Browne erected on the previous centenary surveys the scene. The new work is a great success. Shoppers rest on the granite seats and stools and snack while kids treat them as skateboard obstacles. Two large white marbles are sculpted into a giant eye and a giant brain. Other carvings are egg-shaped, perhaps alluding to Browne's experiments in embryology. Matt Cooper, who runs the market stall nearby selling belts and leather goods, has made himself an informal ambassador for the work. He explains to me that the eye and the brain are placed on a straight line between Browne's house and church, where he lived and where he is buried. The other pieces are set out in a precise quincunx. I had not noticed this. 'People come and have their photo taken standing by the brain,' he informs me.

On the side of a nearby building, a colourful, hand-painted sign

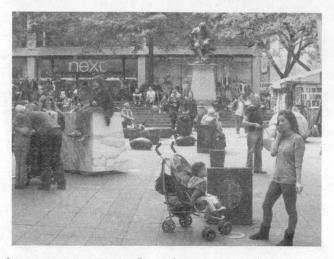

proclaims: KNOW YOURSELF. It is advertising something calling itself 'the human chakra system'. I wonder how Browne would have felt about this appropriation of the Delphic maxim of the modern medical profession. A few steps away is the Body Shop with its absinthe handwash, 'Wild Rose Nourishing Hand Butter', and the Rainforest range of haircare products containing 'pracaxi oil' and 'Community Trade aloe vera' and 'No Silicones'. Would Browne walk past muttering under his breath 'quacksalvers'?

A pall of incense wafts from a shop called Inanna's Festival. The sign on the pavement outside promises: 'Angels Fairies Candles Crystals Green Men Goddesses Glitter & Sparkle. Tarot consultations. Bringing Magic to Life'. The crystals and the Green Men would once have been believed to possess magic powers. Maybe some customers still choose to believe that. But they are not sold with that guarantee. It's only a bit of fun. Everybody is in on the game. It is impossible to take offence at these emporia, surely. Or should they be closed down as irresponsible peddlers of pseudoscience?

I am contacted out of the blue by a man who used to don seventeenth-century costume in order to impersonate Browne – until the day he was mugged for his efforts. Kevin Faulkner was a porter at the Norfolk and

Norwich Hospital, but was made redundant. He now volunteers at the Church of St John the Baptist on Maddermarket, one of the Norwich churches no longer used for worship. Inside, the furnishings are a miscellany gathered together a century ago by an overenthusiastic vicar. There are many older memorials, including an exuberant monument to the Layer brothers, sixteenth-century mayors of Norwich, crowded with marble figures and polychrome emblems, which Kevin is especially proud of.

We swap favourite passages of Browne, and he presses into my hand a Victorian novel by one Mrs Marshall, *In the East Country*, in which Thomas Browne appears. It is a romance involving his favourite son, young Tom, and a beautiful girl who comes seeking aid for her sick father. Browne senior beams paternally over the proceedings but plays no real part in the action. Kevin's interest in Browne was kindled when he read Sebald's *The Rings of Saturn* and has developed into something of a pursuit. He has his own theories about the man, believing that he was a greater follower of the Swiss-born physician Paracelsus than is usually credited, that he was close to Arthur Dee, the son of the noted scholar and alchemist John Dee, and physician to King Charles I, who retired to Norwich, and that he was a follower of the German natural philosopher and collector Athanasius Kircher. Jumping in time, he finds sympathies, too, with the symbolism of the twentieth-century psychologist Carl Jung.

I realize we are pulling in opposite directions. Like some other fans of Browne, Kevin is busy enmeshing him in a network of mystics, 'turning the clock back to the esoteric', as he puts it. I'm trying to wrench Browne into the present. But of course Kevin has tried that, too. I should proceed with caution.

Why is our mutual friend not better remembered? 'He made the fatal mistake that I've made of staying in Norwich,' Kevin tells me. It is curious that Browne was content to remain here after having tasted the intellectual fruits of the continent. In 1668, his son Edward moved to London, became a fellow of the Royal Society and published papers in the *Philosophical Transactions*. But these opportunities had not been available when his father was young and mobile.

Later, I find a recording of Kevin declaiming passages of Browne. He reads with a singsong lilt and pauses to colour significant or unusual words in a way that breaks the run of the prose. The effect is arresting, but it is not the voice of Browne that I have in my head at all.

Was Norwich in fact the making of Browne? In many ways, knowing what we know about him now, it seems the perfect place for him, cosmopolitan but not at the centre, removed from the worst of the disturbances of the time, a place where sceptical and irregular views might be tolerated as long as one didn't make too much of them.

He belongs to Norwich now. He is, as I have said, its most famous son, even if he is adopted. His is the only statue in the city I have ever noticed. It is hard to believe. Is there nobody of incontestably greater stature? A military or political figure who could be forced to fit the heroic mould? An inventor or a poet? There is – so far – not even a statue of Alan Partridge.

Browne first made Norwich belong to him. A physician is able to insinuate himself into the community as few professions can. He became known to the landed families of Norfolk who depended on him for medical attention, and he depended on them to extend his network of contacts with gentlemen-scholars known at the time as virtuosi.

But he also made himself belong in more exceptional ways. He studied the indigenous flora and fauna. He planted in the soil, and from that soil unearthed long buried relics and remains. He found that roots do not just go down. They also spread sideways. Roots are links. The archaeological finds that Browne describes reach back to other cultures – Roman, Saxon, Viking – paralleling his own correspondence with scholars abroad. He finds interest in the local and the particular to complement the worldly knowledge in his library, and it is by finding a correspondence between the two – between his garden flowers and the orchards of a Persian prince, between urns found in a Norfolk field and the funerary customs of the Pharaohs – that his writing gains its rich texture.

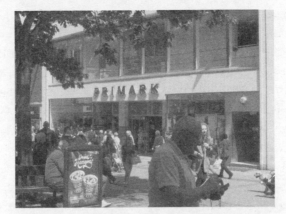

And now he is buried here. His monument is the sign that he walked here once. It is our evidence that he had an attachment to this place as well as the testament of subsequent generations' claim on him. It is not the most reliable evidence, as Browne knew well. In *Urne-Buriall*, he writes: 'The Reliques of many lie like the ruin of *Pompeys*, in all parts of the earth.' But Browne's lie here, between Primark and Next. Everyone is sure of that.

I began this chapter with Thomas Browne's death on the date of his birth, and promised to come back to this 'remarkable Coincidence'. I do so because it is a marvellous demonstration that we still possess the urge to think about Brownean problems in Brownean ways. We still do not know the answer to this particular conundrum, and we do not even know whether knowing the answer would be useful or significant, or just a curiosity.

The most famous person thought to have died on the date of his birth was then, and is still, William Shakespeare. He was born probably on 23 April 1564 – it is known only that he was baptized on 26 April – and he died on 23 April 1616. Browne may have been aware of this or not. The enduring singularity of this one celebrity's tidy departure from the world should give us a clue that birthday deaths are not especially common. But what are the facts?

Modern states keep records of the births and deaths of their citizens. There are the makings of a global database that could surely resolve once and for all the question of whether there is anything statistically exceptional about a birthday demise. The figures might supply evidence to support a hypothesis that disproportionate numbers expire owing to the excitement and overindulgence on the day, for example. Or, conversely, they might suggest that celebrants are so invigorated by the jubilation, or so reluctant to mar the occasion, that they find themselves able to hang on that bit longer to life. More profoundly, is there a wish, conscious or subconscious, to subside into oblivion upon achieving once again this annual milestone and to depart the world with a proper sense of closure?

It is a tempting problem, and it is not surprising to find that a few investigators have made a start on the number crunching. David Phillips, a professor of sociology at the University of California at San Diego, has been examining death days for more than forty years. In the past, he has examined the incidence of death around religious holidays, observing a 'postponement effect' in Jews approaching Passover and in Chinese coming up to the Harvest Moon festival. These particular holidays offer two advantages to the statistician. First, they are moveable feasts and so seasonal and calendrical effects do not distort the analysis. Second, they provide a clear-cut comparison with statistics on non-Jews and non-Chinese who do not observe these holidays. Phillips's observation of 'postponement' – a reduced incidence of deaths leading up to the holiday, and a corresponding spike in deaths shortly afterwards – suggests that some people are indeed able to influence the timing of their death. In 1992, he turned his attention to birthdays, examining the records of 2,745,149 Californians who died of natural causes. He found that women were slightly more likely to die in the week before their birthday and men were slightly more likely to die during the week following. He concluded grimly that 'the birthday functions as a "deadline" for males'.

However, a more recent study of more than 300,000 terminal cancer patients in Ohio contradicts this and other previous research by finding no significant difference in the numbers dying around their birthday or on holidays. These researchers chose cancer patients as the focus of their study in order to eliminate the complication of seasonal variation in the mortality rate – cancer claims its victims all year round, unlike heart and lung disease which peak in the winter months – and also because they thought that people dying of chronic disease over a long period of time would be among those most likely to be able to manipulate the time of their death. Of course, the fact that there turns out to be no observable effect here may simply indicate that cancer is a uniquely callous angel of death, deaf to all appeals for clemency.

New Swiss research looking at national statistics over a forty-year period covering 2,380,997 deaths, on the other hand, claims to have found that an astonishing 13.8 per cent more people die on the exact anniversary of their birth than on other days of the year. Since the increase was observed only among people aged sixty and over, this seems to be a very pronounced effect indeed within this group. The observed effect was approximately equal in men and women, even though women's deaths were ascribed mostly to physical health problems, whereas suicide and accidents were more likely to be the cause in men. In general, the researchers announced, 'birthdays end lethally more frequently than expected'.

David Spiegelhalter, a statistician at the University of Cambridge and professor (for 60 per cent of his time, he says) of the public understanding of risk, is sceptical of this result. It is 'so biased by errors in recording as to be unreliable,' he tells me. He notes that the Swiss figures record the 13.8 per cent spike in deaths without any dip in mortality rate in the days leading up to the birthday or any dip afterwards, effects which would also have to be present if we were to be confident in inferring from the data that some people have the ability to delay or hasten the date of their death. For this reason, and because there is, as the Swiss researchers themselves say, no differential effect at all related either to sex or to cause of death, David believes the blip might arise in fact from a systematic error in the record-keeping. As it turns out, the researchers' apparently significant 13.8 per cent amounts to only 900 persons – that is, 13.8 per cent of 2,380,997 divided by 365.25 for the days of the year. An alternative – and David thinks more plausible – explanation, given this arithmetic coincidence, may be that these 900 souls (who after all comprise only 0.04 per cent of the total sample of 2,380,997) have simply been subject to transcription errors where the official registrar, perhaps mesmerized like Browne by an idea of neater symmetry, has inadvertently replicated the figures recording the day and month of the person's birth in the column for the date of death or vice versa. 'Maybe with better records it will be more studiable in the future,' David suggests.

This is not to say that no coincidental effect should be expected at all. Modern statistical records show that there are broader effects to be considered too, which Browne, with his medical mind, might easily have added in to his reckoning. The major one is the seasonal fluctuation in the death rate owing to winter diseases. The winter of 2010–11 saw a typical number of excess deaths of 25,700 in England and Wales; that is to say, 25,700 more people died during the months from December to March than during the four-month periods preceding or following. Taking into account the whole population and the overall mortality rate, it emerges that people are some 20 per cent more likely to die during the winter. This effect is remarkably constant. In the seventeenth century, when disease transmission was poorly understood and protection against the elements was rudimentary, there was still a 20 per cent increase in deaths in March and April, although a few places, including Norwich, also recorded 'anomalous burial peaks' in the late summer months. This seasonal effect clearly influences *individual* chances: if you happen to have been born in the winter, you are now that much more likely to die on your birthday; if you were born in the summer, you are less likely to die on your birthday by a similar margin.

However, it does not alter the *overall* odds of people dying on their birthday as long as the overall birth rate is constant throughout the year. The problem is, it isn't. Today, the birth rate varies on an annual cycle, governed in part by seasonal variation in fertility but chiefly by when couples choose to procreate. In England and Wales during recent decades, summer births have run at a 10 per cent greater rate than winter ones. When both the birth rate and the death rate exhibit their own annual cycles, then a correlation does emerge, which does distort the overall probability of people dying on their birthday. The easiest way to understand this is to consider a hypothetical extreme case that everybody who dies in a given year dies on one designated day, let's say 21 June. Now, if the birth rate is constant through the year, then still only one person in 365 dies on their birthday. If the birth rate is higher in the summer, however, then the proportion of birthday deaths will be increased simply because that many more people happen to have been born on 21 June. The real population may well exhibit a similar anomaly. Here, if many more people die during the winter *and* mothers give birth disproportionately during the summer months, then the overall odds of a person dying on their birthday will be considerably less than 1 in 365, because so many summer-born people die in the winter. Those born in the winter, on the other hand, are always going to be more likely to die on their birthday than the rest of us so long as we continue to suffer from winter diseases.

It surprises me that uncertainty continues to swirl around Browne's 'remarkable Coincidence'.* For all our databases and computer power, it seems we still don't know whether it is truly remarkable or not if we happen to die on our birthday. Although they may disagree on both the extent and the direction of any effect – towards postponement of death

---

* The 'remarkable coincidence' is fatally compromised if it is true, as Browne told the antiquary John Aubrey, that he was born on 19 *November* 1605. Aubrey had written to Browne seeking biographical material on him, but Browne gave such a meagre résumé of his career that it would not make even the briefest of Aubrey's *Brief Lives*. Had Browne been included, he would have found himself in the splendid literary and scientific company of Francis Bacon, Robert Boyle, John Dee, William Harvey, René Descartes, Thomas Hobbes and Robert Burton. Browne's stature would have been increased. Perhaps, though, he was doing his best to see through his long ago stated hope to make 'a totall adieu of the world'. As for that date, is November an error made in haste or the unwelcome truth? No independent record exists of Browne's date of birth. But in younger days, he had written that the ascendant sign at his birth was Scorpio, which is compatible only with an October date.

or its acceleration – these studies do seem to agree on one thing, which is that some of us at least are able to manipulate the timing of our dying. They invite us to look at dying as a manifestation of human behaviour, not merely an inevitable natural phenomenon. This conclusion would of course come as no surprise to Thomas Browne or to any learned figure of the seventeenth century, who would simply be puzzled that we have had to go to so much labour to believe it.

I happen to mention to some Norfolk friends the puzzles and paradoxes of anniversary dying, and the fact of Browne having fulfilled his own statistical possibility, when they tell me of a woman who went one better, and died on her hundredth birthday. It seems that the woman – the mother of an acquaintance – retired from the celebrations of the day, went upstairs to rest, and quietly expired. A perfect and punctual centenarian. What are the odds?

2

Physic

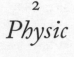

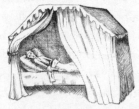

"'tis as dangerous to be sentenced by a Physician as a judge'

Letter to a Friend

IN A PERIOD when outbreaks of plague are frequent and life expectancy hovers around forty years, news of a woman who has reached the age of 102 might be considered remarkable enough. But great age alone is not what draws Thomas Browne to Elizabeth Michell of Yarmouth. He writes to a correspondent in the Royal Society: 'what is most remarkable about her is a kind of boulimia or dog-appetite; she greedily eating day and night what her allowance, friends and charitable persons afford her'.

Browne's short note, 'Boulimia Centenaria', is revealing not so much for what it says about the woman as for what it says about the conduct of **medical** practice. He describes her physical condition – she is 'a person of four feet and half high, very lean' – and her circumstances – she is 'very poor, living in a mean room with pitiful accommodation'. He notes

❀❀❀❀❀❀❀❀❀ ❀ ❀ ❀❀❀❀❀❀❀❀❀

medical (PE, 1646): Relating to physicians or the practice of medicine. New, it is surprising to learn, as an adjective, as in a 'medical man', and a noun, a 'medical' being a preparation of 'medics' or herbal remedies rather than a doctor's examination. Browne uses the word in the preface to *Pseudodoxia Epidemica*, where he manages his readers' expectations of what follows by explaining that it had to be written in moments seized between executing his duties as a doctor. 'In this work,' he warns, 'attempts will her ability to answer his questions as well as her confused belief that her eldest daughter is in fact her mother. He reports her varied diet of 'flesh, fish, apples, pears and any coarse food', adding that 'She vomits not, nor is very laxative.' Although he is drawn to Elizabeth Michell primarily as a curiosity, he acknowledges the reality of her condition, which he calls a 'disease'. In a digressionary footnote, he repeats a story out of Plutarch: did you know that Caesar's assassin Brutus was similarly afflicted with bulimia on his march to the Battle of Philippi? Browne concludes: 'though I am ready to afford my charity unto her, yet I should be loth to spend a piece of ambergris I have upon her, and to allow six grains to every dose till I found some effect in moderating her appetite; though that be esteemed a great specific in her condition.'

It is in its way a thoroughly modern encounter. Browne displays curiosity and compassion. He is alert to a possible connection between the woman's medical condition and her environmental circumstances. The medicine is unusual but like all medicines at this time it is naturally sourced rather than made artificially (ambergris is a fatty accretion ejected from the stomachs of sperm whales and could be found floating on the sea or lying on the coast). Browne has a clear idea of its specific effectiveness, and is aware that dosage is an important factor. He is also conscious that medicine costs money, that he must husband his resources in order to run his medical practice at a profit, and that attention given to a 102-year-old may not in the end be, as today's euphemism has it, optimal resource allocation.

It's easy to see the medicine of the past as insufferably primitive in the light of modern advances. However, although the procedures and remedies may be different, Browne's period bears some striking

---

exceed performances: it being composed by snatches of time, as medicall vacations and the fruitless importunity of uroscopy [the examination of urine for the purpose of diagnosis; another Browne word] would permit us.' In fact, it is the work's great strength that it was undertaken in such routine circumstances, for it is surely this that guarantees its consistent tolerance and good humour.

similarities with today. Then as now, medical practice is pluralistic, and undergoing scientific and social change. There are many folk and traditional remedies, some based on empirical observation, others on no more than superstition. Formal medicine is still dominated by the Hippocratic theory of the four humours and Galen's discoveries in human anatomy. Diagnosis and treatment are based on identifying an excess or a deficiency in the humours – blood, phlegm, yellow bile and black bile – and trying to correct the imbalance. In practice, it is easier to get rid of an excess than to replenish a shortfall. This is done by physical means often assisted by purgative substances likely to produce a desired response – coughing up phlegm, vomiting yellow bile, or passing a black stool. Excess blood is relieved by bloodletting using a lancet or scarification. This system has been refined over two thousand years and is second

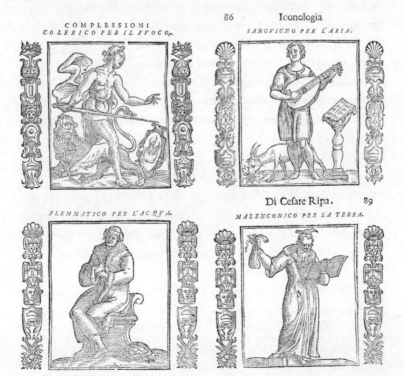

51

nature to all physicians. Although it sounds crude now, it has much to explain its longevity.

The four humours correspond with four temperaments – sanguine, phlegmatic, choleric, melancholic – and with the four elements, earth, air, fire and water. The key sensations associated with them are easy to grasp. They are dry, wet, hot and cold. A combination of cold and wet signifies an excess of phlegm, for example, while the choleric is associated with hot and dry symptoms. Foods with opposite qualities could be prescribed to correct an excess in one humour. Overall, the system is remarkably robust and self-consistent.

But there are the stirrings of an entirely new medicine. Many medicinal plants are documented in herbals, but it is not yet understood that certain chemical constituents within them are responsible for their action. In the sixteenth century, Paracelsus began to investigate combinations of extracts from plants and minerals in an effort to make more effective medicines. He was guided by alchemical principles, and his recipes are therefore not always to be trusted, but his innovations nevertheless mark the beginnings of chemical-based medicine. His ideas spread slowly through Europe, and gradually it is recognized that chemical substances may provide an effective means of controlling disease.

Browne uses saltpetre to reduce fevers, for example, but it is not yet known why it is effective. (It reduces blood pressure.) The difference between various kinds of horn is of concern to Browne, too, especially as quacks are advertising as unicorn horn what is in reality walrus tusk. In fact, all such animal parts may be used as a source of ammonia and ammonium salts, which have many medicinal uses (indeed, ammonia is known as 'spirit of hartshorn'). Nevertheless, it is still thought that the character of a medicine is intrinsically linked to its source in a specific plant or animal. Even chemicals were useless against many diseases, though, such as dysentery and other 'fluxes', smallpox, diphtheria, typhus and whooping cough, all life-threatening illnesses for which we now have effective vaccines.

Other complaints were more manageable. 'The stone' – calculi of the bladder or kidney – was especially prevalent in East Anglia where the water is hard. A stone could sometimes be dissolved. Some of the questions in *Pseudodoxia Epidemica* that might seem merely academic or facetious turn out to have strong underlying reasons for their inclusion. The bizarre belief that a diamond will dissolve in goat's blood, for example, seems hardly worth the answer, but for the fact that it is so important to know more about substances that might soften or break hard substances in order to cure the stone. But surgery was often the only option. In a letter to his son Edward, Browne remarks on the speed of one surgeon, having read in 'our common newesletters, that Sr Arthur Ingram was cutt of the stone that the operation was performed in 3 minutes'.

Outbreaks of the plague are regular, and the signs and symptoms are unhelpfully varied. It does not behave like many minor ailments in line with the humoral system. It is 'the most multi-faceted of early modern diseases', according to one medical historian. It is in cases of the plague above all when physicians fall back on Christians' preparedness to suffer; their own ministrations are of little use.

Diagnosis is not by examination – taking the pulse, listening to the breathing and so on – but relies, as we see with Browne and Elizabeth Michell, on visual and environmental clues. The colour and pattern of skin under the fingernails is one key to revealing an excess of this or that humour. The environmental context is not only the circumstances in which the patient lives, but also the sky he or she lives under. Doctors routinely use astrological methods to inform diagnosis and to give out prognoses. This is not quite the desperate resort it might seem. In ancient Greece, Hippocrates had sought to relate medical conditions to the constellations as a means of ensuring that his teachings could be universally applied – a seasonal illness had a connection to the seasons and so did the stars. An astrological association functioned as a kind of international shorthand when identifying diseases. It also helped the patient, allowing them to relate their illness to the world around them and to shift blame for it away from their own sinfulness. Today, we invoke environmental and genetic factors to perform the same function. The historians Ole Peter Grell and Andrew Cunningham believe that 'the career of astrology in English medicine points to a loss that is still felt and expressed in various ways, such as noncompliance and resort to alternative medicines and nostrums'.

The range of medicines seems odd to us today. They come from natural sources – animal, mineral and vegetable – the unsurprising topics of the first three books of *Pseudodoxia Epidemica*. Lapis lazuli is a (hugely expensive) purgative. Bezoars (hairballs or other concreted matter found in the stomach) are an antidote to poison. Coral is said to be effective against epilepsy. Lapis judaicus (not a stone but the shelly parts of certain sea urchins) is a diuretic. Though some regard them as poisonous, Browne instructs that mistletoe berries be taken for purgation. Some people today use mistletoe preparations as a cancer therapy. This would seem to be a classic example of an unapproved alternative 'medicine'. But the idea has been taken with sufficient seriousness that clinical trials have been conducted, although they have so far proved inconclusive.

These medical substances are ranked by efficacy. The first group amounts to little more than recommended foods. Substances active in the second degree are those that produce an observable humoral effect. Those in the third degree (from which we gain the still current figure of speech) have a more violent effect. This hierarchy is as it was in Hippocrates's time. The major difference in the seventeenth century is that there is now a broader range of first- and second-degree substances available so that the severest remedies are less often required. The repertoire of such medicines continues to expand apace, encompassing everything from powerful prescription painkillers to vitamin pills and spot cream.

Browne, it is perhaps surprising to find, emerges as something of a campaigner for modern medicine. Like many of today's practitioners, he dismisses ancient medicines if they do not exist in some modernized version. 'It is folly to find out remedies that are not recoverable under a thousand years,' he writes in *Pseudodoxia Epidemica*. By this, he eliminates the classical remedies of Aristotle and Pliny, Hippocrates and Galen unless they have been ratified by the learned men of the Renaissance, much as a modern doctor will shun a herbal remedy but happily prescribe a commercial pharmaceutical based on the same active ingredient. But he is not likely to prescribe a radical dose of some chemical if he judges that a moderate alteration of diet might prove just as effective. He is disdainful of a growing tendency to commercialism in medicine, which has produced some bizarre sideshows, such as the ransacking of Egyptian mummies for supposed medicinal material, owing to confusion with a prized Persian oil known as 'mummia'.

Though death comes early and often, there is a rudimentary idea of preventive medicine. Each spring and autumn equinox is the time for pre-emptive purging of noxious humours by bloodletting. Interest is growing in the role of diet and exercise. It is noted, for example, that those who perform physical labour eat and sleep better than the idle rich. The 'air' is seen as important to health. 'Such as is the air, such be our spirits', notes Robert Burton in *The Anatomy of Melancholy*. He lists many places tainted by bad air, including Lynn in Norfolk, although John Evelyn makes a point of noting the clean air of Norwich. The merits of different meats are debated. Browne is part of the discussion, considering why we regard only certain animals as food, and even broaching the idea of vegetarianism: 'there is no absolute necessity to feed on any'. It is an advanced view – Evelyn was an enthusiast, too. A vegetarian diet will not become popular until Victorian times. As with the vegetarian societies that arose then, Browne's argument is Christian as much as medical. The Bible implies that before the flood, when people seemed to live to far greater ages, man subsisted entirely on herbs and fruit: 'to you it shall be for meat'. He does not recommend this scriptural vegan diet, but he does recommend we overcome custom and habit and sample a wider variety of both plants and animals for our own nutrition. As for alcohol, he recommends Christian moderation, but is not against occasionally drinking enough wine to produce a 'sober incalescence'.

The statistic of life expectancy being no more than forty years blurs the truth. Many who die – such as five of the Brownes' children – die in infancy or early childhood. Most who survive to adulthood can therefore expect to live on into their fifties or sixties and beyond. This is a demographic difference that we do not appreciate today when nearly 90 per cent of us can expect to reach the age of sixty. Browne feels that the wide range of ages at which he sees people die must be evidence of a divine hand at work.

Today, we feel we have a clearer idea of our rightful natural span, and that if we fail to attain it, it will be down to some medical cause. But it does not occur to Browne that gaps in medical knowledge play a part, just as I am sure it does not occur to my GP that some as yet unforeseen advance might lengthen the odds against my dying when he thinks I will. And it may well come. I am distracted to find that the records kept by the Office of National Statistics do not merely show a continuing decrease in age-standardized mortality (the rate at which people die in a population standardized to reflect the actual range of ages in that population), but a decrease that is exactly linear. The graph line slopes downward from about 1,300 deaths per year per 100,000 of the male population and 800 deaths per year per 100,000 of the female population in 1960 to 700 and 500 per year per 100,000 respectively in 2010. At this rate, well before the end of the century, we should all be living for ever.

The national health is a free market. There are a few charitable hospitals – Norwich is lucky to have one. Everybody else pays. Medical practitioners are both licensed and unlicensed. The unlicensed ones aren't necessarily worse than the licensed. 'Herb women' are often preferred for their 'more constant and easy cures than learned physicians', according to the natural philosopher Robert Boyle. Fees for a simple treatment such as a vomiting or a bloodletting might be a shilling, as much as a weaver, say, might earn in a day. Empirics sell cheap medicines – at best filling the role of today's pharmacies, at worst palming off the sick with useless or dangerous substances.

The medicinal function of many herbs or 'simples' is common know-ledge, and so people also make up their own remedies. Homes had no medicine cabinet, but a well-equipped household would have a battery of equipment for the routine preparation of medicines – sieves, mortars, syringes, cupping glasses, decoction pans. These traditional methods stand in contrast to the exotic concoctions of the apothecary. It is a choice that is hard to comprehend today when all that we once knew about the curative power of plants seems to have been lost. Because of this ignorance, and because there are also poisonous plants, and because the dosage is crucial, our modern doctors warn us off this kind of self-medication. Before chemical medicine, though, the 'cures' expen-sively prepared by the best physicians were often only thinly disguised versions of commonly available remedies – although part of that thin disguise might be an important judgement about the dosage. The herb women may be hardly more reliable – they are surely also the 'old wives' of old wives' tales and Browne's pseudodoxies. Yet the welcome they receive should warn us how rash and terrifying the modern notions of a male physician could appear.

Browne is practising when physicians are just beginning to sense the new power they have over their patients. They know it is not only the dose but also the way in which substances are ground and prepared that is critical to their effectiveness. Men with continental training under-stand that 'foreign remedies', widely feared as poisons during the wars of the late sixteenth century, may in fact be superior to traditional English cures. Like Browne they guard this professional knowledge, devoting some energy to the denouncing of *Saltimbancoes*, *Quacksalvers*, and *Charlatans*'.

The medical beliefs and practices of any era seem ignorant and brutal to the ages that follow. In this, medicine is distinct from science, for we esteem scientists of earlier generations and say that we stand upon their shoulders, yet we laugh at the sawbones of the past.

I am inclined to turn this conventional view on its head, if only to see what happens. Let us stop being rude about early modern medicine

– its humours and leeches, its bloodletting and vomits – and think more about our own doctors. How much confidence should we place in them? It is a strange case of faith. These professionals stand before us in panoply – with special premises, distinctive tools, obscure jargon. We are in no position to judge the veracity or quality of what they tell us. We have little choice but to trust their advice. To modern physicians we are like the unquestioning religious faithful were to their priests in previous centuries. This is not to say we should disbelieve them. Often they are in possession of the skills and tools to repair our health – but then so were, if perhaps less often, the physicians of Stuart England. What we should understand is that there are always good doctors and bad doctors, effective and less-effective medicines, specific and general remedies, medical conditions that are well understood and medical conditions that are hardly understood at all.

Today's profession is not without its own foibles. I am obliged to visit my local GP's surgery when I am laid low by an acute stomach bug. I see a doctor who is neither my registered doctor nor, unfortunately, the doctor I usually see on my infrequent visits, and who I once managed to importune, since he looked already extremely relaxed, on the subject of Thomas Browne, at a drinks party. I am out in under ten minutes clutching a prescription for some opioid that will address my symptoms and a mild bewilderment at the doctor's lack of curiosity about the cause of my illness.

The doctor suggested that he could prescribe some antibiotics, but has left it to me to point out that with no infecting bacterium identified, this would be unlikely to be effective (and, I don't add, possibly irresponsible, given that the indiscriminate prescribing of antibiotics is a chief reason for their growing ineffectiveness). He asked me if I would like a referral, but again has left it to me to ask what for. At the end I feel as if I have been played, and that he has had me labelled all along as one of the 'worried well'.

I dutifully take the pills, of course, each one reminding me of the sway that the pharmaceuticals companies have over the medical profession.

I wonder how Browne would have regarded my experience. He would have been interested to witness the brief physical examination by the doctor and intrigued as to what my blood test could reveal. He would have been struck, I think, by how incurious the doctor is about me, by how few questions he asks about my habits and diet. He might have been puzzled at the doctor's reluctance to explore possible causes of my illness and simply prescribe medicine for the symptoms. He might even have noticed that this may be what prevents a more revealing discussion taking place. Nevertheless, he would have been impressed by the efficient way this was done – and by the fact that my consultation was free.

The problem clears up a few weeks later of its own accord. I had turned down the doctor's offer of an antibiotic, and can imagine that had I left the GP's surgery and sought out a homoeopathic remedy I might now be gaily ascribing my 'cure' to this. For isn't this how homoeopathic medicine 'works', through our getting better anyway?

The modern patient understands the deal. The drug is a conciliation, or more precisely a propitiation, a gift of appeasement. It appears to offer a solution, completing a transaction in which the patient has confided their symptoms and the doctor has given something in exchange. We have talked ourselves into a position where this suits everybody. Prescribing a drug, even something useless or inappropriate, is quick and easy for the busy doctor, it gives the patient the appearance of a cure, and of course the surgery may be making money from the drug company by doing it. There is no equivalent of this business in Browne's time when everybody knows that medicines are derived from herbs.

For a different view, I turn to Anna Waldstein, a modern 'herb woman'. An ethnobotanist at the University of Kent, she wrote her doctoral thesis on Mexican migrant workers in the United States, who often avoid professional medicine and rely instead on traditional remedies. 'And they are healthier than middle-class American citizens,' says Anna with a laugh. For most of us, though, this useful knowledge has been lost. 'We think of medicines as rare things found in the jungle, but the reverse is almost the case. Many common plants with medicinal properties grow by pathways and in areas disturbed by people.' As our ignorance has grown so has our suspicion of these plants, tacitly encouraged by the food and pharmaceutical industries, which have brainwashed us into reliance on commercial products. But Anna believes the tables may turn, as it is realized that our health services are built on an unsustainable business model. Already we are being urged to greater levels of self-care. With NHS endorsement, this idea could be revived. Anna would like to see 'a primary care herbal medicine kit with five or ten really established herbal medicines, for things people want to self-treat anyway, like indigestion'.

We should not romanticize the seventeenth century. Then only the rich could afford a doctor, and medicines were by and large less effective. But we should at least try to understand that there were positive aspects as well as negative ones, that Browne's medicine was advanced for its time, and that the delicate gamesmanship of doctor and patient went on then as it does now.

Even so, in the reign of Charles I England was no centre of excellence in medicine. Even at Oxford, the tutors encouraged their graduates who wanted to pursue a career in medicine to complete their studies abroad. Leaving England in the summer of 1631, Browne was to spend the next three years at Europe's leading medical universities. A year at Montpellier was followed by a year at Padua and a year at Leiden. Each place had strength in a different field. Montpellier was a centre of botany and pharmacy, Padua was at the height of its fame in anatomy, and Leiden was where Browne was able to bring together medicine, natural history and philosophy with a practical ethos that would equip him for his professional life.

Thanks to his father's bequest, these places formed a major part of Browne's education. The university cities prized their tolerant attitude to other peoples and religions. The long and difficult journeys between them, however, bore witness to the upheaval of the Thirty Years War between the Catholic and Protestant powers of Europe.

Montpellier became a Protestant city during the French Reformation, something for which it has still not been forgiven by the time Browne arrives, nine years later. It is rebuilding after a siege by the Catholic forces of Louis XIII, and simultaneously recovering from a severe outbreak of the plague. François Rabelais studied and taught medicine here in the previous century. His riotous, inventive prose will inspire some of Browne's more unlikely literary adventures. Rabelais's contemporary Guillaume Rondelet was professor of medicine and a pioneering naturalist, whose treatise on marine animals becomes a frequent reference work for Browne. Browne would almost certainly have also enjoyed direct contact with Lazare Rivière, a Paracelsian proponent of chemical medicine, Pierre Richer de Belleval, the father of modern botany and keeper of the first botanical garden in France, and the university chancellor François Ranchin, a specialist in childhood diseases who distinguished himself by his stoical management of the outbreak of plague in 1629.

Browne has time to explore the countryside plants and animals. He picks up the langue d'Oc to add to his other languages. Somewhere the silk merchant's son is beguiled to witness the 'strange and mysticall transmigrations' of silkworms; they turn his 'Philosophy into Divinity'.

At Montpellier, it is not the plague, which has claimed 2,000 lives, that captures his medical interest. He observes a disease he has not seen before, which the locals call 'morgellons'. Much later in life, he recalls seeing these cases as he allows himself to wander off-topic after making some remarks on the semiotics of beards:

> Hairs which have most amused me have not been in the Face or Head, but on the Back, and not in Men but Children, as I long ago observed in that Endemial Distemper of little Children in *Languedock*, called the *Morgellons*, wherein they critically break out with harsh Hairs on their Backs, which takes off the Unquiet Symptomes of the Disease, and delivers them from Coughs and Convulsions.

It might have amused Browne further, or perhaps horrified him, to learn that 'morgellons' has been reinvented for the twenty-first century.

Early modern physicians had made sporadic reports of the symptoms – eruptions of hairs or worms, nobody's really sure which, on fleshy parts of the body – in the past, although Browne is the first to record the name 'morgellons', the name which stuck, and which is now making a dramatic return. Recommended treatment is by heating the skin, or the application of milk, honey or fat to ease out the hairs, followed by shaving or plucking. Leeuwenhoek's new microscope could find no source of animal infestation, however, and by the end of the seventeenth century 'the vogue of worms' was in decline, notwithstanding the occasional spectacular resurgence, as in 1791 when a Leipzig physician wrote that 'cinder-coloured animals may be made out, having two horns, round eyes, a tail which is long, forked, with the extremities, which are bent up, covered with hair. These worms are terrible to look at.'

In 2001, Mary Leitao, from Peters Township a few miles outside Pittsburgh, Pennsylvania, found that her two-year-old son, Drew, had developed sores on his lip. He complained of a strange feeling under his skin, and reportedly used the word 'bugs' to describe it. His mother noticed what were apparently small fibres emerging from a few of the sore spots. Several, and soon many, doctors could find no satisfactory explanation for what was wrong with the child, although some prescribed creams for eczema and scabies. Eventually, one doctor, again finding nothing wrong with her child, dared to suggest to Leitao that she should see a psychologist.

As it happens, Leitao had a degree in biology and had worked as a hospital laboratory technician. She tried another course. She searched online and found Browne's description of morgellons. She launched a campaign, the Morgellons Research Foundation. Soon, others were coming to her with reports of similar symptoms. Some had tried desperate measures to rid themselves of the sensation of worms under the skin. Gradually, her campaign gained supporters and momentum. It was covered on television, and still more sufferers came forward. The

Morgellons Research Foundation eventually reckoned that 12,000 people made themselves known. In 2006, driven by public pressure, the Centers for Disease Control and Prevention, the United States government body in charge of public health, set up a task force to investigate the disease. It examined a representative sample of 115 sufferers in northern California. The CDC report found material collected from the study subjects' skin was mostly cellulose, probably from cotton clothing. 'No parasites or mycobacteria were detected.' Another study, by the Mayo Clinic, examined a similar number of patients. Neither institution could trace any consistent infection or environmental cause. Both concluded that the symptoms were consistent with a condition known as delusional parasitosis in which patients only *feel* that they have an infestation.

These days, though, a dismissive report by government-nominated scientists is no longer likely to be the end of the matter. It merely serves to stir conspiracy theories. After all, how can a delusion also have physical signs – the hairs or 'bugs' that many patients had collected, which did not seem to them to be harmless cotton fibres? Surely it is an unreasonably dedicated patient who goes to the trouble of harvesting actual hairs and presenting them as evidence. A government would have every reason to suppress information concerning an uncontrolled outbreak of

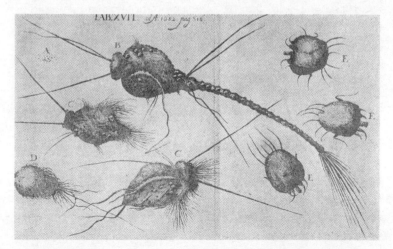

a new disease. Its secret activities might even be the cause: undisclosed environmental leaks, untested new nanotechnologies, and the 'chemtrails' of chemical or biological weapons seeded into the atmosphere by military planes have all been proposed as explanations for morgellons.

It is harder to accept that you might have a mental disorder as opposed to a physical one. The latter is your bad luck, the former is your weakness, is the view we know others will take. American dermatologists faced with patients claiming to have morgellons were advised to acknowledge their patients' suffering, and to accept their use of the word 'morgellons', but then to prescribe antipsychotic drugs and to treat their condition as a delusion.

Who owns morgellons? Certainly not Thomas Browne any more. Many Internet sources now claim that morgellons is an entirely new disease, as named by Mary Leitao. Some even say that it is a new name for delusional parasitosis. The name and its ownership matters as an assertion of patient power. If sufferers can persuade their physicians to use the name too, then it shows they have won a small victory over government authority. A segment of the medical profession acknowledges the right of patients to call their illness what they like even as they prescribe them antipsychotic drugs. Others resist acceptance of morgellons at any level. So it becomes another reason for people to distrust doctors. And at the bottom of it all, in America, is the matter of medical insurance. For the insurance companies to accept that morgellons is a legitimate condition, so that victims could claim the cost of treatment against it, would be the real victory.

Writing this, I begin to feel quite itchy myself. It is easy to see how this 'disease' spreads. It is a meme, not a virus. You only have to come into contact with words describing it to start feeling the symptoms. It is therefore extraordinarily susceptible to self-diagnosis. Epidemiologists talk about the vector of a disease, meaning the living agent that transports the pathogen so that the infection spreads. In the case of the plague, the vector is the fleas that live on rats. The principal vector for malaria, commonly known in Browne's England as the 'quartan ague', is the mosquito. In the case of twenty-first-century morgellons, the vector is the Internet. Without the Internet, people would never have been able to compare notes on symptoms and even swap photographs of their own irritated skin with such rapidity that a few cases could multiply to become a phenomenon.

How is a meme-spread disease distinguishable from a disease spread by virus or bacterium if both have symptoms and signs? Are they any different at all?

I am inclined to side with the modern medical profession. After all, which is more likely: the feeling that our body is infested with some kind of parasite, or the eruption of actual hairs that can be traced to no identifiable natural or synthetic source? I wonder if the availability of handheld microscopes that connect to your computer also has something to do with the proliferation of morgellons. It is curious that the hairs that characterize the disease seem to have got smaller since Browne's time, when microscopes were not available.

But I am sympathetic to the plight of morgellons victims. Whatever is imagined, their suffering is clearly real. How ought doctors to respond? A British GP I know has not heard of morgellons by name, but has no trouble recalling an occasion when a patient came to him complaining of morgellons-like infestation. He asked the man if he could produce a specimen of the parasite. A stool sample from the patient was sent for testing and found to contain an earthworm that the patient must have placed there. I can imagine the doctor's exasperation at this time-wasting, and hope he did not let it show. Perhaps he felt it was a desperate cry for attention, itself in need of medical help. It may be right that Mary Leitao has now closed the Morgellons Research Foundation, but it is surely not right that her name now appears in an online 'encyclopedia of American Loons'.

Shakespeare in *The Taming of the Shrew* praises 'fair Padua, nursery of arts'. A city of the Venetian Republic, in the seventeenth century Padua and its ancient university had a custom of ignoring papal decrees and welcoming in Protestants, Jews and Muslims as well as Catholics. Here Galileo taught for fifteen years before moving to Florence and running into trouble with the Pope for his views on the solar system.

For Thomas Browne, Padua was the centre for the study of anatomy at a time when it was becoming important for physicians to understand the architecture of the human body. A knowledge of anatomy would promote understanding of the true cause of mysterious diseases and inform diagnosis.

Portraits and busts of great names in Renaissance medicine now line the walls of the Palazzo del Bò, the historic university building. In the sixteenth century Italians such as Bartolomeo Eustachi and Gabriele Falloppio, who gave their names to the Eustachian tubes in the ears and the Fallopian tubes that connect the ovaries to the uterus, were joined by anatomists from all over Europe. Greatest of all was the Flemish Andreas Vesalius, or Andries van Wezel, who assumed the university chair in anatomy on the day of his graduation in 1537 at the age of twenty-three. His masterwork *De Humani Corporis Fabrica* became the standard textbook on human anatomy for Browne and for many generations afterwards. John Caius, Browne's distinguished medical

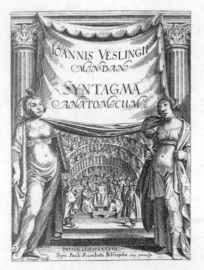

predecessor in Norwich, went to Padua to learn anatomy from him. William Harvey graduated from the college in Cambridge that Caius went on to found, but also obtained his doctorate in medicine at Padua. His work on the circulation of the blood, *De Motu Cordis*, was the first notable breakthrough in physiology by an Englishman. It was published – abroad – in 1628.

It was Harvey's teacher Girolamo Fabrizio, known as

Hieronymus Fabricius, who constructed the first permanent anatomy theatre in Padua. Previously, anatomical demonstrators had relied on ad hoc arrangements, even performing dissections in the street. Fabrizio's design, which still survives, though much altered by restoration, has six steeply tiered balconies where students can stand to gain a clear overhead view of the dissection which takes place on a central table. A story I have heard that a canal running directly under the demonstrator's table allowed fresh cadavers to be floated in and dissected remains to be flushed away turns out to be a myth. It is nevertheless an eminently practical design and it became the prototype for anatomy theatres around the world.

I look among the surrounding shields and portraits for any commemoration of Browne's year here in 1632. But there is none, and the guide has never heard of him.

All anatomists at this time were conscious that they were following in the footsteps of their classical predecessors, Hippocrates and especially Galen. Many, such as Caius, regarded Galen as being without fault. Vesalius was a more judicious admirer. Some of the things he saw in the body during the course of his own dissections did not agree with Galen's writings, and he was not afraid to say so. Browne's position was more nuanced. It suited him in his later writing to present himself as more traditional, or antiquarian, than he really was. He certainly would not have wished to appear in print to be overriding the classical masters of his profession as Vesalius was happy to do. Browne refers to Galen frequently but never to Vesalius, though after his time in Padua he was fully apprised of recent advances.

Browne's final year abroad took him to Leiden, another stronghold of academic freedom and tolerance. He matriculated at the university and gained his medical doctorate in the same month, December 1633, although it is likely that he spent some months here before and after.

I've been looking for a place that evokes the seventeenth century so that I can immerse myself in Browne's period. I feel it's not just the historical fabric that must be more or less intact in order for me to do this. There needs to be an atmosphere and an attitude of mind that infuses the streets, some expression of the fact that there have been religious wars, hardships survived, riches accumulated, connections made with the world. I'm looking for evidence, too, of awakened curiosity and the new spirit of enquiry.

Norwich does not have it. The architecture is too mixed – medieval, Victorian, modern – and the people teeming in and out of the chain stores are too firmly located in the now. Oxford is too unreal. Padua seems to have its heart still further back in time, reflecting the earlier start of the Renaissance.

But I find what I am looking for in Leiden. It is quietly prosperous, discreetly learned, a civic success. The brick houses are respectable and modest. A cat is asleep in the picture window of a furniture restorer's workshop, the image of industry and domesticity.

In the Museum Boerhaave, I find some of the medical teaching aids of the time: alarmingly realistic wax models of opened human bodies and anatomical atlases in which you can peel away layers of skin and flesh simply by turning the pages. I stand in the anatomy theatre, which

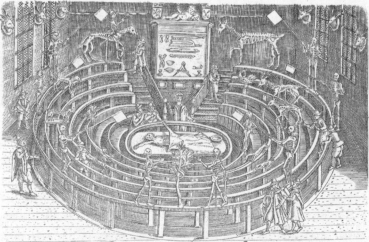

THEATRUM ANATOMICUM.

has been reconstructed from seventeenth-century engravings. Above me dangle animal and human skeletons, including a complete man on horseback, and banners proclaiming 'Mori ultimum. Vita brevis' and NOSCE TE IPSUM.

Leaving Leiden, Browne returned to England accomplished in many languages. He was qualified in the disciplines of medicine, anatomy and physiology, and the sciences of botany and chemistry. At Leiden he had seen how this knowledge could be used in following a career fully engaged in civic life and yet still allow for the pursuit of the curious. He had experienced a variety of customs and mores in other countries that had taught him the virtue of tolerance. Browne had acquired an awareness of difference, and knowledge that what is to be found in one place – a plant, an animal, a disease, a variety of religion – may be absent in another, and that there is no deep moral to be drawn from this.

Norwich could boast of nineteen physicians in the decades before Browne settled there, the largest concentration outside London. There was a medical practitioner of some sort for every 200 citizens. But there was no adequate hospital. A modern hospital would not be founded until 1770, and the charitable religious house known as the Great Hospital of St Giles, founded in 1249, was in temporary decline. It has rebounded since as a retirement home and so upholds its claim to have been in continuous use for more than 750 years. When I visit orderlies are rushing back and forth with food for the kitchens. An old man waylays me and asks excitedly: 'Did ye see the noo buildens?' They are very fine. But the old building that still stands among them gives a fair idea of the basic level of medical provision. The one ward is a long upstairs room above what was once a chapel. It is divided like a stable so as to give each patient some privacy and a Gothic arch through which to watch the world go by.

Aside from physicians and unlicensed herb women, there were also the barber-surgeons. The abundance of hairdressers in Norwich today barely hints at the gruesome past of that trade when men who cut hair and trimmed beards were also licensed to let blood, pull teeth and attempt major surgical operations. Only the red-and-white barber poles serve as a reminder – a stylized image of bloody bandages. With heavy heart, Browne would when necessary have referred his patients to the least disreputable of these.

But it might not come to that. Thanks to his continental training, Browne has enviable expertise. He augments his current knowledge of the field with continued reading and observation throughout his career, and is able to employ what he has learnt for the benefit of his patients. All this ensures he remains at the forefront of medical practice. He implicitly accepts Harvey's theory of the circulation of the blood, and sees its wider implications. For example, he notes the effect of alcohol, transported, as he correctly presumes, in the bloodstream, on the brain. He deduces that medicines, too, might prove efficacious on parts of the body far from where they are introduced.

Rickets is identified in 1645, and is investigated by a working party of the College of Physicians in 1650. Browne recognizes that the condition is unusually prevalent among the children of East Anglia and speculates on its causes. Rickets is a softening of the bones owing to a deficiency of vitamin D, which the body obtains chiefly from conversion of choles-terol in the skin by ultraviolet light from the sun. This of course was not known then, but Browne presciently believes that sunlight may be a factor – he recommends it should be investigated whether 'Children of the English Plantations' suffer from it, too. (Rickets has made an unwelcome return in the twenty-first century, the unforeseen conse-quence of people using sun-blocking creams in order to reduce the risk of skin cancer – and, supposedly, also of children spending too much time indoors playing computer games. Hospital admissions increased four-fold between 2001 and 2011.)

Browne's reputation is soon established in Norwich and the county beyond. He rides out to visit wealthy clients at Oxnead and Raynham and Gillingham and Crostwick. In April 1644, soon after Browne is established in his professional practice, Thomas Knyvett of Ashwell-thorpe, chides his wife for calling a doctor from eighty miles away:

'meddle no further with Phissick with out an Apparant necessity and the Advise of Dr Browne, for heer is no further direction to be had'. Towards the end of his career, in 1678, Robert Paston, the earl of Yarmouth, writes to his wife, Rebecca, with encouraging news about their friend: 'My Lord Townshend has had a severe fitt of the gount [sic] & stone both together or rather the strangurie, butt as I heare was left somewhat better on Friday by Sir Thomas Browne who was sent for to him.'

Such notes of admiration and relief are typical. A few clients are even moved to praise Browne's skill and discretion in verse, one man whose wife was suffering from an unknown disease telling 'How with exactest care, / Hee's thoughts of her distemper did declare'.

Browne is conscientious enough to feel guilty taking his fee when he has effected no cure – but he takes it anyway. He is aware that people in general put too much faith in physicians' powers of diagnosis and cure. He acknowledges their propensity to make false connections between cause and effect. Large parts of *Pseudodoxia Epidemica* are concerned with correcting such medical misapprehensions, but it is my guess that he bites his tongue when a patient offers his own wild opinion of where his disease has come from. Most doctors learn to judge character so that they can tell if a patient is likely to refuse medication or won't change his habits in order to improve his chances of recovery. Browne is unusually attentive to such factors for the period. He is firm with patients, such as Hamon l'Estrange, who wishes to try a remedy that has worked for a friend of his, but which Browne assures him is unsuited to his weaker constitution. He is also considerate over how he breaks the news that a patient has a potentially fatal disease.

Inevitably a large part of his job is to attend patients who are dying or who are racked with pain, which he can do nothing about. Often they are children. The first year of life is so dangerous that 'we scarce count any alive that is not past it', Browne writes. On one occasion, he has to inform the Paston family that two sons 'could not live to be men' and another 'was so sickly that he was [not] likely to live a yeare'. Seeing 'the thousand dores that lead to death', he thanks God 'we can die but once'. He will not offer false comfort, but he knows the effect it has to tell a patient that 'he is at the end of his nature'.

The actual moment of death is ascertained by using a feather or mirror glass to confirm the cessation of breathing. Browne laments that it is not his profession's custom at this time to record the cause along with the age of death. Today we cannot die without being given a 'cause of death', no matter how decrepit we are. Modern practice expresses a medical materialist view that death is a kind of defeat, that the body is like a machine that has broken and on this occasion cannot be repaired. This in turn promotes the impression that death is an avoidable accident rather than the ultimate fact of our lives. It is a sad truth today that at the end of life you are liable to be regarded more as a medical failure than as a dying human being.

The American surgeon and writer Sherwin Nuland reports that present-day physicians often withdraw when there is nothing more they can do, less out of respect for the patient and their loved ones than out of disgust at the ultimate professional setback they have suffered and their own horror of death. It is, he suggests, their way of recognizing that 'the real event taking place at the end of our life is our death, not the attempts to prevent it'. Medicine's humility in the face of natural death has been replaced by embarrassment. It is a shift that Browne would have surely regretted. When he died himself, the cause of his death was not recorded, only, as we have seen, the gentle manner of it, 'like a wise old philosopher'.

Browne's acceptance of the inevitable at whatever age it comes, and his exceptional care and sympathy for both his patient and his patient's loved ones at this time, is movingly recorded in one particular case from the middle of his career.

Robert Loveday of Chediston in Suffolk was a traveller, translator and would-be poet. He died of tuberculosis in 1656 at the age of thirty-five. An engraving by an artist named Faythorne shows him to be uncommonly handsome, with a straight nose, steady gaze and luxuriant curled hair tumbling down to his shoulders. There is the hint of a thin moustache on his lip. A verse underneath the likeness records:

> Loveday, thy feature here by FATHORN drawn,
> Though it display his Master-piece of Art,
> It cannot represent the smallest grain
> Of those clear rays of thy diviner part,
> The Royal fancies of thy loyal heart.

Loveday was precocious, diligent, kind and modestly ambitious, though always sickly. He also possessed a rare power to affect those with whom he came into contact. It seems that he suffered with phthisis, as tuberculosis was then known, for some years. Early on during the disease's rampage through his body, Loveday wrote: 'I confess I do more than suspect a Consumption, and if that be designed to fetch me from this World, I think I shall go without reluctancy; for I have already received enough of the Divine hand to make me admire his bounty: but I have fair hopes of a recovery.' Yet he must have known for a long time that he was destined to die of the disease. Meanwhile, he and his family did what they could for his health. He was taken away to Bath for the waters, then brought back for the healthier air of East Anglia. He grew painfully thin. He exhibited the cruel symptom of late-stage tuberculosis sufferers that they believe themselves to be in extraordinarily good health. He dreamed beautiful dreams. As his condition worsened, he called for Thomas Browne, who was known to the family. Although Browne was twenty-five miles away in Norwich, a day's ride distant, it was he 'from whose advice I fancy most hope of all'. But it was already far too late. When Browne at last sees the patient, he gives him only months to live. However, he continues to visit him, charting his weight loss, and monitoring the change in his appearance: 'I never more lively beheld the starved Characters of *Dante* in any living Face'. He has the opportunity to observe his decline right up until 'his soft Departure...so like unto Sleep, that he scarce needed the civil Ceremony of closing his eyes'.

Browne records Loveday's final journey in a document now known as *Letter to a Friend*. Much of it was composed as Loveday lay dying and shortly after his death. He kept the draft and added to it and polished it nearly twenty years later, although the finished version was not published until 1690, after Browne's own death. It is a curious melange of bedside reportage of Loveday's deteriorating physical condition, more general clinical notes, acute psychological observation and epidemiological speculation. Infusing it all like a balm is a paean to Loveday's person that Browne extends into a universal manual of virtuous living. The eponymous friend is believed to be Sir John Pettus of Cheston Hall in Chediston, a natural philosopher and politician, who was not present at the house when Loveday passed away.

It is certainly no ordinary note of condolence. The commingling of the pathological and the poetic makes for odd, even uncomfortable, reading. The death of Robert Loveday is described with compassion, even beauty, but unsparingly and without sentiment. Browne does not say the glib things we say now when someone dies: that the suffering will pass, that we will 'get over' it, or even, as we might expect from a true Christian centuries ago, but which is still reheated in secular desperation today, that the two men will be reunited in some afterlife.

Cold fact and high praise meet in the very opening sentence, where Browne tells Pettus that Loveday is both 'Dead and Buried, and by this time no Puny among the mighty Nations of the Dead'. The physician cannot forbear to set the death in a brutally honest context: 'considering the incessant mortality of mankind', he writes, Loveday is just one of perhaps a thousand people who have died in the same hour (an underestimate, in fact; the daily global death rate must have been in the high tens of thousands in the mid-seventeenth century; the hourly death rate due to tuberculosis alone at this time might be several thousand). He goes on to give a visceral description of his last days, 'his Flesh being so consumed that he might, in a manner, have discerned his Bowels without opening of him'. A reader of entrails, he adds, might almost read the man's fortune through his skin.

More is to follow in regard to the unenviable predicament of the physician in the face of incurable diseases, and we should not be surprised also to find a defensive note of self-justification creeping in as Browne places on record his gentle discouragement of unrealistic hopes for recovery. He knows that, in the seventeenth century, ''tis as dangerous to be sentenced by a Physician as a judge'. But he does as he must. He tells the family that Loveday has only months left to live or, as he poeticizes it for the wider intended readership of the *Letter*: 'he was not like to behold a Grashopper, much less to pluck another Fig' – that is, he might see the summer but not another autumn.

Browne naturally witnessed many deaths, from newborn infants to the very elderly, and including several of his own young children. What makes Loveday's special? First of all, it is a 'good death', that is to say one with which the Church could be satisfied that the dying person was fully prepared for the afterlife, as codified in the fifteenth-century Latin texts of the *Ars Moriendi*. This preparation would cover personal composure, vestments, religious ceremonies, Bible-reading, family attendance and valedictions, any and all of which might be jeopardized if death came suddenly. Loveday's 'soft Departure, which was scarce an Expiration' is good also in the sense that he appears not to be suffering at the last, something that is far from commonly the case.

Loveday has furthermore prepared for this eventuality with great personal sacrifice, announcing that he will not marry or have children. But he does not give up the mental fight, remaining outgoing, receptive and generous:

In this deliberate and creeping progress unto the Grave, he was somewhat too young, and of too noble a mind, to fall upon that stupid Symptom observable in divers Persons near their Journeys end, and which may be reckoned among the mortal Symptoms of their last Disease; that is, to become more narrow minded, miserable and tenacious, unready to part with any thing when they are ready to part with all, and afraid to want when they have no time to spend.

His young age is a problem, of course. Browne finds ingenious ways to rationalize it. Is Loveday not, for example, the equal of an old man from whom have been deducted all the days he 'might wish unlived'?

Browne so admires Loveday's example that he seeks in *Letter to a Friend* to develop it into a model for all, though it is hardly a realistic path for many to follow. The perfect but truncated life of Loveday is implicitly set in moral opposition to the continuing flawed life of his friend Pettus, for whom Browne appends a series of recommendations for personal conduct, which he reuses as the basis for his last work, *Christian Morals*. This 'how to live' guide is a companion piece to Loveday's object lesson on how to die. But it is a cloying list: 'Tread softly and circumspectly', 'pursue Virtue virtuously', 'let not disappointment cause Despondency', 'Be charitable before Wealth makes thee covetous', 'Triumph over thy Passions' and so on. Pettus was only eight years younger than Browne, and it is not clear he would have welcomed the advice. It is perhaps as well that Browne's son Edward saw to it that *Letter to a Friend* was only published some years after Pettus's death.

Browne surely sees himself – a younger, less fortunate version of himself – in Loveday. Like Browne, Loveday is well travelled, a linguist and a writer. He has an ambition to study medicine, if letters to his brother are to be believed. His declaration that he is ready to leave the world having 'already received enough of the Divine hand to make me admire his bounty' chimes with sentiments often expressed by Browne. Browne's extraordinary sympathy for Loveday's plight is surely ignited by his identification with their shared creative sensibilities and moral outlook.

Browne is accepting – not frustrated or angry, not even resigned, but accepting – in the face of an incurable disease, such as Loveday's consumption, because it is God's will. It is not yet usual to view a mortal illness as an affront or a challenge to medical science. Robert Bayfield, a younger Norwich contemporary of Browne, wrote in a medical treatise of 1655, *Enchiridion Medicum*, that there was similarly no 'general method of cure' for the plague because it was God's 'rage'. Pain and illness were part of God's plan, either as salutary messages to improve our moral behaviour, or as reminders of our own impending death and the hereafter. Browne acts as God's messenger in spelling this out to Pettus.

But perhaps the early death of the paragon Loveday shakes his certainty in this. For it is not entirely constant in his attitude that acceptance is the only option when life is threatened. Suddenly, he is thinking more in the way our doctors think today, when death is a sign of professional failure, but it is a surprising view in the seventeenth century when God takes man when He is ready.

3
Animals

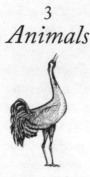

'The world was made to be inhabited by beasts'

Religio Medici

'I SEND YOU THE scull of a poulcats...Probably you have none by you.' Most of us get by well enough without having the skull of a polecat to hand. That Thomas Browne regards such an item as essential – and his blithe confidence in this letter to his physician son Edward that he will regard it so too – is entirely in his character as a student of nature and as a collector of miscellaneous objects. As an article of correspondence between the two Brownes, this is not untypical. Thomas has succeeded in transmitting his passion for the curiosities of nature to his son, for in his dwellings in Salisbury Court off Fleet Street in London Edward also keeps an ostrich. The father is concerned for its well-being and writes on another occasion: 'I beleeve you must bee carefull of your Ostridge this extreme cold weather least it perish by it being bred in so hot a countrey and perhaps not seen snows before or very seldom.'

Thomas Browne is not what we would call now a nature lover. His interest in animals is dispassionate; he can see and accept that man, too, is part of nature. This makes him gently critical of Christian doctrine, which demands little cognizance of the natural world even as it grants man dominion over it; he is more admiring of 'the Heathens' in this respect. So he is seldom to be found watching birds in their habitat. More often, he has specimens brought to him, dead or alive, and he is just as likely to record the taste of a bird as its appearance. Young herons are sometimes served at feasts, but the bittern, he notes, 'is also comon & esteemed the better dish'. His engagement with nature is coldly scientific, by modern standards even cruel. At one point, he kept an eagle, which he fed on puppies, cats and rats, but did not water, probably as part of an experiment concerning the flesh of certain birds such as the peacock, which might be preserved indefinitely in a dried state for food.

There are expedient reasons for Thomas – and Edward – to be able to distinguish the skull of one species from that of another or to recognize a sweet flag or a cicada when he sees one. The correct identification of animals and plants is essential when they are used as sources of medicines. There are also signs of divinity to be decoded in God's creation. But chiefly, I feel, it is for the sheer pleasure of knowledge that Thomas describes the natural riches he finds around him.

Notes and Letters on the Natural History of Norfolk is a partial catalogue of birds and fishes (including a few aquatic mammals) to be found in the county and its waters. It was not conceived as a book by Browne, but was assembled posthumously from letters written to Christopher Merret, a physician and one of the founding fellows of the Royal Society, who was preparing a complete natural history of England. Browne's list is not exhaustive; the species chosen must be those that most interested him or that he thought would be unfamiliar to Merret in London.

The project placed Browne in a classical tradition he was familiar with. He often cites the natural histories produced by Aristotle, Claudius Aelianus and Pliny the Elder – despite this last work being the original source of many of the 'vulgar errors' concerning the natural world that Browne seeks to set right elsewhere. Their medieval and Renaissance successors, the thirteenth-century German friar Albertus Magnus, and later the Bolognese naturalist Ulisse Aldrovandi, the French traveller Pierre Belon and others, produced volumes that were progressively more complete and more reliable. Such work laid the foundations for

Linnaeus, whose Latin binomial system of naming plants and animals at last established order and eliminated confusion between species described in different languages.

Browne's ambition was more modest – to describe the local species in a way that others would find helpful. Even so, he was making an important new kind of record. The *Natural History of Norfolk* gives English names to the *shearwater* and the *merganser* for the first time. He also names the *mistle thrush* from the berries it feeds on. From well beyond the coasts of Norfolk, he appropriates from Scandinavian languages the name of the *narwhal*, which features in his lively discussion of the existence or otherwise of unicorns in *Pseudodoxia Epidemica*. Other creatures he gave common names to range from the expressive *praying mantis* to the minimally described *red spider*, which later science has shown not to be a spider at all but a species of mite.

Browne's investigations into the natural world ran well beyond the naming of species, however. He was greatly interested in how animals came into the world, and investigated the ways in which eggs responded to various substances with such scientific thoroughness that he earned the praise of Joseph Needham, a later pioneer of chemical embryology. He was the first to use the words *amphibious*, to describe creatures that live both on land and in the water, as well as *oviparous* and *viviparous* (meaning egg-laying and giving birth to live young, respectively).

It is hard in these days of images transmitted in an instant to recapture the sheer hunger for knowledge that has Browne prepared to ride across the county in order to see a beached whale or send a man out into the marshes with a shotgun in order to bring back the corpse of some rare specimen for display or dissection. We are accustomed to having our nature delivered to us with less effort – the drive-by nature of a raptor glimpsed from a car window, the packaged nature of hour-long television programmes. We sit on the sofa imbibing the sweet concentrate of the BBC's *Springwatch* rather than stepping outside the back door.

I have a regular walk that I take when I feel I have earned a break from work. It is a loop of three miles or so with habitats as varied as

can be managed within the narrow limits imposed by the Norfolk topography. It begins down the loke by the side of my house, which leads to
the edge of a soggy riverside pasture. I follow the fields that border the
river, where the farmer has given his grudging consent to my presence,
still mistrustful of anybody on his land for whatever reason. I cut across
another piece of rough grazing land, then onto a country road over the
river, past well-tended gardens, through a churchyard, and over the river
again, this time on a warped wooden footbridge, and back along the old
railway path. If I am lucky I don't see another person.

I call it the twenty-five-bird loop. It is not a study on the scale of
Gilbert White's parish of Selborne in Hampshire. Nor is it quite Charles
Darwin's 'sand-walk' around the little wood he planted at his house in
Kent, where he made circuits that gave him time to think. Twenty-five
species of birds seen during the hour or so the walk takes me is par for
the course. I see more on a cold day, and would see more still if I permitted myself to go first thing in the morning. I see fewer birds if it is windy,
as it often is, or if it is a hot afternoon. The varied habitat helps boost
the count, and so does the fact that most of the walk runs along edges
– edges between land and water, between cultivation and wildness – for
it is at the edges where animals prosper, able to shuttle quickly between
food and shelter.

I have built up a rough expectation of what I will see where as I make
my circuit. The same nest sites and roosts are used year after year. I am
beginning to be able to predict the days of departure of the swifts and
swallows and the arrival of the fieldfares and redwings. It is not a walk
made for rarities. I am mostly content to see the ordinary pattern repeat
itself with minor variations. But of course there have been exceptional
sightings. Briefly, one bitter winter's day, three whooper swans rested on
the bare field. Another time, a marsh harrier swooped across it looking
for a service-station snack en route between the reed beds of the Broads
and the north Norfolk coast. I have seen the rare water rail and, once, the
even rarer red-backed shrike – a male in full plumage perching in full
sunlight. I waited for it to do the shrike's thing of skewering an insect

on a thorn for later consumption, but it only emitted repeated creaking noises, waiting for me to go away.

I also observe what crops go into the fields, what chemicals go onto them, and what contestable vermin the farmer has been shooting. I do not have in my house the skull of a polecat, but I do have the skull of an American mink, whose body I found one day on this walk, having been executed marksman-style neatly shot through the head.

Browne chose his county well for natural history. Norfolk is a large county with a very long coast that bulges out into the North Sea. It is the first landfall for birds windblown from the east, and its mudflats and marshes provide rich winter feeding grounds for geese, ducks and waders. Browne's global sensorium – his lofty view of the world – is in evidence once again, since he is one of the first naturalists to insist that many species are annual migrants, a realization that must surely have come from observing large flocks moving along the Norfolk coast in the spring and autumn months. Some birds land so exhausted on the coast that it is possible to take them with dogs or simply to club them to death, he reports; they must have flown long distances over the sea to arrive in this sorry state. Until the idea of long-distance migration was accepted more than a century later, people believed, in one of the greatest of 'vulgar errors', that swallows, for example, hibernated at the bottom of ponds.

Though Norfolk is famously low-lying, it is nevertheless rich in habitats, including forest, fen, marsh, saltings and wetland as well as grazing fields and arable land. Much of this environment, and especially the shore, is not much changed from what Browne knew, although today the positive effect of managing coastal habitats for wildlife is countered by the intensive agriculture that prevails inland. For this reason, the species noted by Browne that are no longer common are birds of the inland heaths now turned to prairies of barley and sugar beet.

The most recent edition of Browne's *Natural History of Norfolk* that is not part of a collected works was published in 1902, and carries a knowledgeable introduction and footnotes by a local ornithologist named

Thomas Southwell. These comments provide a useful interpolation between Browne's century and our own, whereby we can trace the long-term progress of many local birds. Some that were relatively common are barely clinging on – the stone curlew, one of those species of the inland heaths, that was 'still far from rare' in 1902 is now quite definitely rare. Even the starlings, which Browne found 'remarkable in their numerous flocks', are now so diminished in numbers they can hardly muster a murmuration.

Other species have undergone a more complicated change in fortunes. Browne describes the avocet, with its smart white-and-black plumage and upturned bill – 'so that it is not easie to conceive how it can feed' – as 'not unfrequent' in the Norfolk marshes. But Southwell's footnote describes it as 'another bird which formerly frequented the marshy districts of Norfolk at the breeding time, but which has now been lost to us', not seen since 1818, he adds, their feathers apparently much prized by fly-fishermen. Today, though, the avocet is once again quite common year-round, the apt symbol for the campaigning success of the Royal Society for the Protection of Birds. At the RSPB's Titch-well nature reserve on the north Norfolk coast there is a path to one of the hides that is dug out like a First World War trench so that visitors will not disturb the birds and the avocets swoop extravagantly about your head as you walk along it.

The *Natural History of Norfolk* does not count as one of Browne's great literary achievements. It is little more than a list of kinds, with each given just enough description to make identification unambiguous. But it gives us a little context as to why particular species were valued and how man saw himself in relation to them; Browne often includes a note that jars with us today as to a creature's likely fate. Knots, huge flocks of which still gyrate like wafts of smoke over the low-tide sands of the Wash in winter, are netted and then fattened by candlelight for the table, for example. Rooks are sold in Norwich market, their livers used in the treatment of rickets. And 'Godwyts [are] accounted the dayntiest dish in England.'

Things have changed. We no longer eat these birds. We now consume them visually. Yet this altered relationship to the natural world is just as pathological in its way. The short bestiary that follows is drawn from creatures that Browne lists in his natural history or that he discusses in *Pseudodoxia Epidemica* because people once believed foolish things about them. It describes the creatures themselves, but it becomes a dissection of how we see nature now.

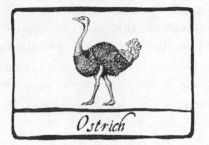

Ostrich

The avocet is the logo bird of the RSPB. But I have noticed that in Norfolk the ostrich vies with it as an emblematic presence. There is such a number of Ostrich Inns that you might suppose the bird once ran across the open heaths of the county in search of liquid refreshment. When I asked local people about this, nobody was able to explain it, and they seemed never to have noticed the signs. I eventually traced the motif to a story involving the Norfolk-born Sir Edward Coke, who became the admired attorney general of Elizabeth I (appointed over Francis Bacon) and James I, and whose family seat was later at Holkham Hall. He adopted the emblem of an ostrich with a horseshoe in its beak, a cliché of medieval bestiaries. As a lawyer, it seems he identified with this creature that was reputed to be able to digest the hardest things. To the ostrich, there is nothing especially significant about iron. The bird is merely looking for hard stones for its gizzard, and as an exceptionally large animal it is able to swallow large pieces which might well include nails and even fragments of horseshoes.

To start with, Browne is inclined to discredit the belief that an ostrich will digest iron. In *Pseudodoxia Epidemica* he confesses he has not had the opportunity to do the experiment; instead he cites his preferred ancient authorities, such as Pliny and Aelian, who make no mention of such a curious habit, but surely would have done so if they had known of it, and others who have refuted the tale by experiment, such as Aldrovandi, who witnessed an ostrich ingest iron but then spit it out again.

Long after the last edition of *Pseudodoxia Epidemica* has been published, Edward Browne, by now a physician at the royal court, acquires one of the birds, from a flock given to Charles II. Thomas is eager for Edward to tell him all about it: whether it tucks its head under its vestigial wing to sleep, whether it is attentive to disturbance in its environment like a goose, whether it is terrified of horses or avoids bay leaves. And he suggests that his son puts to the test the willingness of the bird to digest iron – perhaps he should wrap a piece in pastry as an inducement. The results are not on record.

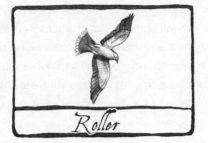

Roller

On my birthday I learn that a roller has been spotted in the unappealing environs of the Edgefield dump near Holt. Thomas Browne was
the first to record a roller in the British Isles. On a loose sheet of paper
included with his letters to Merret he notes: 'On the xiiii of May 1664
a very rare bird was sent mee kild about crostwick wch seemed to bee
some kind of Jay.' He describes its glorious plumage in detail – 'violet',
'russet yellowe', 'azure', 'greenish blewe', 'bright blewe', 'the lower parts
of the wing outwardly of browne inwardly of a merry blewe' and other
shades of blue. A Latin name *Garrulus Argentoratensis* has been added
in a different ink and pen at a later date once Browne has had a chance
to locate the name assigned to the bird by Aldrovandi. But he calls it a
'Parret Jay'.

I have only seen one once before, in southern France, but I have a
vivid memory of its appearance from the bird books of my childhood,
where it formed a dazzling triptych with the hoopoe and the bee-eater,
making something like a colour insert among the pages of tweedier
common species. The bird has been there a week by the time I hear of
it. Apparently, thousands of twitchers have responded to their alerts and
have descended en masse in their 4x4s. I realize now that this explains
why a field that is normally empty has been full of parked cars. But I did
not guess the reason in time, and so I have not seen the bird.

I am not one of this breed. I rejoice to spot a rarity on my walk or in
my garden, but hardly any more than I do to see a conspiracy of long-
tailed tits skittering through the bushes ahead of me on a winter's day
or a yellowhammer singing from the top of a tree. I disapprove of those

people who keep pagers and are prepared to tear across the country on news of the sighting of some exotic 'accidental'. We have no true perspective on the cost of our actions in relation to nature, and nor did Browne. The hoopoe, or 'Upupa or Hoopebird so named from its note' he calls 'a gallant marked bird wch I have often seen & tis not hard to shoote them'. Which is, of course, one reason why it is now a rare thing to see a hoopoe in Britain.

Edgefield dump is a blight on the landscape, casting plastic bags far downwind when a gale blows and always leaking a stinking miasma, which can be seen pouring through the chain-link fence around the site. It is also an attraction for birds. A few years ago, a glaucous gull joined the thousands of other gulls wheeling over the refuse, and this too brought in the twitchers. This year, I have noticed a single red kite there – the first I have seen in Norfolk. It is a joy to watch, one of the few birds that can give the gulls flying lessons, fanning and dipping its tail to make extravagant course corrections seemingly just for the fun of it. Common in London in Browne's day as scavengers, although less so in Norwich, where Browne tells us they were outdone by the ravens, kites were lost from Norfolk by the 1830s and almost wiped out from Britain as a whole through the twentieth century. However, an astonishingly successful programme of reintroduction begun in 1989 has seen the kite population increase almost eightfold since 1995. In the Chilterns, they now swarm like pests. Nobody has yet brought back the ravens.

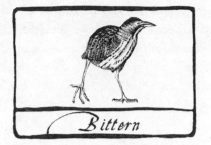

Bittern

Bitterns are not susceptible to rapid-response birdwatching. They are not gaudy and they are not exotic foreign guests. They are, on the contrary, extraordinarily well camouflaged and extraordinarily particular about their habitat – large freshwater areas of common reed. A single male's territory may cover as much as twenty hectares of this kind of land, and this makes it a characteristic bird of the Norfolk fens, marshes and broads. Nevertheless, bitterns were locally extinct by the mid-nineteenth century. They began to make a tentative recovery in the early twentieth century when the first nature reserves were created, but then went into decline again because of pollution and boat traffic. Now, numbers are slowly climbing again thanks to closer management of habitats and even the costly creation of new inland areas of reed bed which will not be vulnerable to saltwater contamination in the event of storm surges and rising sea levels.

I never knew the bittern until I came to Norfolk, and even then it was some years before I saw one. At first, I only heard them. Their sound is universally described in bird guides as 'booming', which suggests a stentorian bird. But on the rare occasions when it has reached me across a Norfolk marsh, it has always been a softer, almost subsonic permeation of the air, like a distant foghorn, or the sound made when blowing across the neck of an empty bottle. Browne describes how Norfolk people believed this 'mugient noise, or as we term it Bumping', was made by the bird using the reeds among which it lived, presumably by blowing them like a bassoon. The delightfully onomatopoeic 'mugient' is another of Browne's gifts to the English language, taken from the Latin verb *mugire*, meaning 'to bellow'. He sought to disprove the story by keeping a bittern in the yard of his house in Norwich. He denied it reeds, but the bird, perhaps lovelorn in any case, never made a sound.

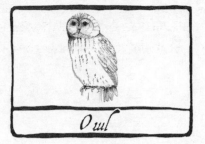

Owl

Our interventions in the name of conservation are well meaning but often clumsy. Barn owls are another species which have made Norfolk a relative stronghold. Browne points out that owls, along with ravens, have long been regarded as 'ominous appearers', associated with Roman auguries. But I have always been happy to see an owl. A night-time drive of even a few miles without an owl – barn, tawny, little – is a disappointment. More often, because roadside verges make good hunting grounds, I see a few, and can estimate the extent of their territories, which are even larger than the bittern's.

In Norfolk, however, the barns where they often prefer to nest have usually been converted into human homes. Following the exhortations of the RSPB, I built an owl box and positioned it low in a large beech tree, carefully oriented in the correct direction. I cut away low branches that might impede the flight path of any bird that wished to take up residence. But I never saw an owl use it. Later, the tree died and stood bare for a year or more before it was felled by a January gale. Inspecting the damage, I found a barn owl crushed in the wreckage of the box. Perhaps I had helped it survive a few winters. Perhaps I had only hastened its death.

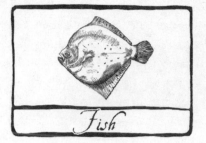

The fish of the sea are harder to catalogue for they live 'in an element wherein they are not so easily discoverable'. Browne prefaces his own list by stating his conviction that the number of kinds is very great – Pliny surely came up short when he stopped at 176 species. But even he cannot believe species numbers are so great that many of them are yet to be discovered. We know now that Browne, while wise enough not to pluck a number from the waves, was still highly conservative in his guesswork. We are always apt to take what we know and assume we know it all. There are 221,000 known (eukaryotic) species in the sea according to the World Register of Marine Species, a figure that is subject to magnification when new discoveries are made, as well as to trimming when it is found, as it quite often is, that a single species has been going under several different names. Furthermore, by looking at the rates of discovery within different animal groups, scientists are able to use statistical methods to estimate the overall number of species yet to be found. According to the latest calculations, for every known marine species there are still ten more waiting to be identified – more than two million species in all.

Browne's list reflects the sea as a larder: mullet, gurnard, plaice, sole, turbot – 'the great Rhombus' – mackerel and herring, the staple of Yarmouth, 'Lobster in great number about Sheringham and Cromer from whence all the country is supplyed', 'Crabs large & well tasted found also in the same coast', oysters, mussels, cockles, clams and 'sea starres', whose five-fold symmetry he celebrates in *The Garden of Cyrus*. '[O]ur starres exceed not 5 poynts though I have heard that some with more have been found about Hunstanton and Burnham,' he comments.

In common with other naturalists of the age – Pierre Belon's illustrated *Histoire naturelle des estranges poissons marins* of 1551 is his principal guide – Browne is happy to lump all aquatic animals together as fish. His list to Merret includes the first Norfolk record of a common dolphin, although he notes that porpoises are commoner. Both are, of course, mammals. When King Charles II visits Norwich in 1671, Browne anatomizes one of the animals, and Dorothy makes 'an excellent savory dish of it'. Seals are so abundant they may be 'often taken sleeping on the shoare'. The seals – common and grey species – were clubbed to death on these shores as recently as the 1960s, but today they bask complacently on the sand in increasing numbers and their pupping has become a tourist attraction during the Christmas holidays. They are mostly left in peace, and their human admirers are watched over in turn by enthusiastic volunteer wardens.

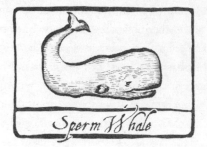

Sperm Whale

When a sperm whale is washed up on the beach at Wells, Browne is quickly on the scene. His alacrity on these occasions forces me to admit that he would probably be among the pager-users today. He finds a sixty-two-foot creature with a peculiar head projecting over its mouth. It has teeth – 'the largest about two Pound' – but no baleen, the bonelike bristles that some whales use to filter food. He recounts the bare fact of the event and others like it – another large whale at Hunstanton twenty years before, and nearby, on another occasion, a pod of eight or nine whales, two of which calved on the shore – in the *Natural History of Norfolk*. But the sensational detail is reserved for *Pseudodoxia Epidemica*, where the stranding gives him the opportunity to investigate at first hand the great mystery of spermaceti.

The spermaceti, after which the sperm whale is named, has long been suspected not to be the sperm of the animal. But as to the true nature and purpose of this buoyant, inflammable and valuable substance, nobody really has a clue. Browne goes to the beach out of curiosity, but he is also interested in obtaining his share of 'that medicall matter', for the substance is esteemed in the making of ointments. It is likely he has competition in this. The scenario is one we know from prints made by Dutch artists. Jan Saenredam's 1602 engraving of a whale stranded at Beverwijk shows armies of sightseers advancing on the unfortunate beast, and some even clambering on top of it. In similar prints, people have brought buckets to take away the precious fluid.

Browne inspects the whale as closely as the stench permits. 'Out of the head of this Whale, having been dead divers days, and under putrefaction, flowed streams of oyl and Sperma-Ceti; which was carefully taken up and preserved by the Coasters. But upon breaking up, the Magazin of Sperma-Ceti, was found in the head lying in folds and courses, in the bigness of goose eggs, encompassed with large flaxie substances, as large as a mans head, in form of hony-combs, very white and full of oyl.' He takes samples. He roasts some of the flesh and more oil runs out. But other investigations must be forgone. 'Had the abominable scent permitted, enquiry had been made into that strange composure of the head, and hillock of flesh about it,' he writes. He wishes he could have examined the bladder, the sphincters of the spout, and the 'seminal parts' so that the spermaceti oil at least might be positively distinguished from the actual semen.

Three centuries later, things are not much clearer. Browne's successor in these enquiries is Malcolm Clarke of the Marine Biological Association in Plymouth, who made a lifelong study of these creatures and their fabled rivals, the giant squid, having obtained his introduction to his subject after the Second World War as a government inspector of the British whaling fleet. Clarke has proposed that whales use their reservoir of spermaceti to control buoyancy, altering its density by controlling the

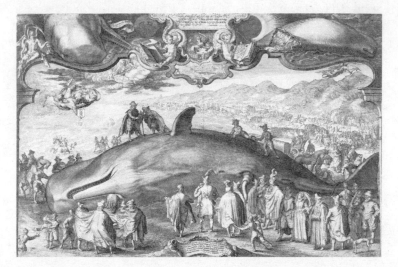

temperature, using water taken in through the whale's spout to cool the spermaceti to make it denser when diving, and increasing blood circulation to warm it again for surfacing. Others believe that the spermaceti acts as a medium assisting in echo location.

Another Norfolk stranding occurred on Christmas Eve 2011: a sperm whale, some twelve metres in length near the Le Strange Arms at Old Hunstanton. After a couple of days, somebody stole teeth and part of the lower jaw using a chainsaw. By New Year's Day, the animal had become an attraction for walkers, its jaw half sunken in the sand with a pool of bloody water nearby. There was a large gash in its side from which some fibrous material was escaping. Well-dressed people stood around in clusters as in the Dutch prints. They kept a respectful distance and took photographs. It is thought that the animal was already dead when it was washed up, as there were no signs of struggle. The local authorities decide the body will be left to be washed out to sea on the next spring tides. By the time I get there after the festivities all trace of the creature has been removed. There is not even a mark on the sand where the carcass lay.

The Dutch regarded whale strandings as ominous. The margins of Saenredam's engraving list a number of further omens and disasters visited upon the Netherlands in the months after the Beverwijk stranding. Whale strandings continue – about 500 cetaceans (whales, dolphins and porpoises) might be washed up on British beaches in a typical year – although today we draw subtly different conclusions from this portent. The whale is no longer an emblem of the grounded ship of state or of squandered riches. We read a different loss, the loss that we are inflicting upon nature, and the loss that this in turn threatens to inflict upon our own species. The vast, ungainly mammal, crashing blindly round the planet, is us.

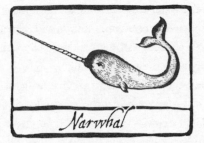

It is alarming at first to find Browne conceding 'there be many *Unicorns*'. He means it literally, though – animals with a single horn. The singular name cannot safely be limited to a single creature of a 'constant shape'.

The problem is that the horns tended to travel without the bodies. They were prize exhibits in the best cabinets of curiosities. Varied in size and colour to suggest that they might originate in many species, they did not conform to the outline of any known animal. The narwhal, which is the rightful owner of a straight, spirally extruded ivory mutation of a tooth, was not fully described until 1685. An inhabitant of Arctic waters, it was an animal that no European but the most intrepid explorer was likely to see alive.

It is understandable that entire creatures are extrapolated (rightly or wrongly) from dislocated parts where those are all that is available. In *Wonderful Life*, Stephen Jay Gould shows how even qualified scientists can be misled. In the early twentieth century, the paleontologist Charles Walcott painstakingly pieced together a range of likely looking shrimps, worms and trilobites from fossil traces found in the 530-million-year-old Burgess Shale of British Columbia. Sixty years later, a new team was prompted to re-examine Walcott's results, and found that he had been insufficiently imaginative. Using new evidence, they rearranged the pieces into fantastical new creatures that did not easily fit within the conventional taxonomic groups. One of these was named *Hallucigenia*, so improbable did it seem, an inch-long monster with a row of seven dorsal tentacles and seven pairs of sharp cones (not unlike unicorn horns in their proportions) which might be legs. Even this may be wrong.

Gould considers the possibility that this assemblage might one day prove to be just one complicated part of a larger organism. And in fact, since *Wonderful Life* was published, new research has suggested that *Hallucigenia* should at least be flipped over, making its tentacles the legs and its legs into spines. Either way up, like the unicorn, it serves its purpose. 'We need symbols to represent a diversity we cannot fully carry in our heads,' Gould writes.

Browne sometimes surprises us with his readiness to credit the existence, at least on some level, of animals we know to be entirely fabulous. Creatures like the griffin, sphinx and chimera he dismisses on the grounds that, like some of the Precambrian creatures of the Burgess Shale, their body parts do not seem to belong together. But the flying horse of Pegasus, the basilisk and satyrs he welcomes because their 'shadowed moralities requite their substantial falsities'. In other words they are too useful to the stories in which they appear to let them go. In an inconsistency not untypical of Browne, harpies are both discredited as being too improbably cobbled together (they have women's bodies but birds' wings, tails and feet), and allowed to 'exist' because of their story value.

His predisposition to reason is in constant battle with his love of the fabulous. After pages discussing whether elephants' legs are jointed (he deduces that they are, on grounds of comparative anatomy, even though their broadly cylindrical shape has led many to believe otherwise), we find this: 'That some Elephants have not only written whole sentences... but have also spoken...we do not conceive impossible.' Not impossible? That elephants *speak*? The story seems to get in because he finds it in Pliny. In a footnote, he adds that the elephant's speech was brief: apparently it said: 'Hoo, hoo.'

It was the Greeks who were responsible for the rumour of the unicorn, which was given scientific authority by Aristotle, who described a kind of ass with a single horn. Pliny was more careful – 'It is astonishing how far Greek gullibility will go,' he writes in *The Natural History*. He based his unicorns on beasts that were at least normally horned, the oryx and the ox. And now at last I can begin to understand how this mythic creature could have grown out of such realities. For among the roe deer that from time to time wander up under cover of the barley to help themselves to the contents of my garden, I occasionally see a young stag with a single antler.

Browne's difficulty is with the version of the animal that has become stylized in emblems and heraldry. The unicorn was incorporated into the royal coat of arms under James VI of Scotland after his succession to the English throne in 1603. It is on my British passport still. The judgement between what is real and what is fabulous is not easy to make at a time when pictures are automatically credited as true in the way that we once thought photographs were. New tales of strange animals from the Americas, made stranger no doubt by inventive retelling, add to the confusion and to the possibilities. Browne points out, rationally enough, that this unicorn would have great trouble feeding if its horn were as long and angled forward as shown in these pictures. But he is on dangerous ground because the unicorn has the force of biblical truth as well as classical authority behind it. It is to be spotted nine times in the Bible, named but never properly described. There is a vague implication that the creature is special in some way, and in Numbers there are references to its great strength, which suggests a rhinoceros or a mutilated ox. But there is nothing more exact. Even the single horn passes without comment.

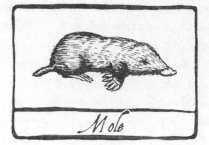

I find it a curiosity – one that Thomas Browne might very well have noted – that the mole seems to seek the air above ground when it dies whereas we seek burial in the earth. For occasionally I find a dead one lying on the grass that does not appear to have been attacked by my cats or any other predator. It happens in early summer after dry weather when I would expect them to burrow deep in search of earthworms in moister soil. One morning, I pick up one of these black corpses for closer examination. I find I can peel back the short, soft fur to expose the skin of the head. I uncover the ears, where tufts of fur adhere more tenaciously, but as I work my way down the conical snout, I find no eyes – merely a hint of dimples where eyes ought to be.

This puts me at odds with Browne, who states: 'that they have eyes in their head is manifest unto any, that wants them not in his own'. I am ashamed at my poor science and hurt by the uncharacteristic tetchiness in my hero's tone. It is apparently a 'vulgar error' to believe that moles are blind. Reading on, though, I am somewhat heartened. Browne's usual authorities are split on the subject. Aristotle finds eyes but no sight, Pliny and others neither eyes nor sight, Aldrovandi, eyes that see. Two centuries later, Darwin proposed that moles' eyes are reduced 'and in some cases quite covered up by skin and fur'. This may be a modification arising out of disuse like the diminutive wings of the flightless dodo, as well as a consequence of natural selection, eyes being positively disadvantageous underground where they would be subject to inflammation from foreign matter entering them.

Modern science remains divided on this ancient question. 'The facts are **incontrovertible** – moles are blind,' the science writer Peter Forbes asserted bravely in 2009. They do, he says, retain the genes necessary for eyes to develop, showing that they have evolved from sighted ancestors. But the results of behavioural experiments in the 1960s suggest otherwise, indicating that although their corneas may be degraded, they do have functioning eyes able to distinguish between light and dark. Apparently, the European mole has open eyes (although you could have fooled me), whereas the Iberian mole has permanently fused eyelids, but in neither animal, according to more recent research, is there evidence that the ocular apparatus is on its evolutionary way out, and it seems that both species are able to detect light and colour. In fact, moles seem to have found ways of avoiding blindness that might be used to address human loss of vision due to corneal and lens defects. He that wants sight in his own eyes may yet have cause to thank the mole.

---

incontrovertible (PE, 1646): Browne employs this word in a meditation on the death of Aristotle. According to legend, Aristotle drowned in the Euripus Strait in the Aegean Sea. Frustrated that he could not understand its ever-changing currents, he threw himself in, exclaiming: 'If I cannot grasp you, then you must claim me.'

Browne does not want to believe this story largely for sentimental reasons. His hero has taken a desperate step, far out of proportion to the analytical defeat he has suffered, for Browne notes that on other occasions Aristotle happily went along with 'high improbabilities', such as the idea that birds dwell in the sun, where they gain their colours. Why, if he felt unable to resign himself to their complexity and mystery, did the great philosopher not just think up some equally fanciful explanation for the tangled Euripus currents? From his desk in Norwich, Browne puzzles over the currents himself. How complicated can they really be? Finding no discussion of the problem in Aristotle's works, and no reliable description of the geographical feature in his classical sources, he begins to doubt their existence at all. The story depends on the supposed fact that the tide ebbs and flows many times in a day, and this, Browne concludes lamely, 'is not incontrovertible'.

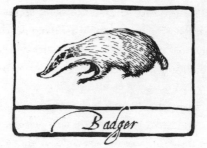

One cool May afternoon, doing my loop, I see a badger in broad daylight on the long eyot between the ditched field I am walking along and the river. It is as startled as I am, and bustles quickly off into the nettles.

The badger provides a precis of Browne's method when tackling vulgar errors. People believed that 'a Brock or Badger hath the legs on one side shorter then of the other'; this was an opinion 'perhaps not very ancient' yet 'very general', Browne tells us. The story was based on observation of what the poet John Clare would later call the badger's 'awkward pace', followed by wild rationalization as follows: badgers, though lumbering, were seen to be able to run in straight lines along the furrows of ploughed fields, and the only way they could do this was if they were adapted to it by having legs shorter on one side.

Browne uses his full armoury of 'Authority, Sense, and Reason', 'the three Determinators of Truth', to deal with the problem. Authority goes first. However, he finds that while Albertus Magnus believes it, Aldrovandi does not. (It is remarkable that these rural myths hold sway across a continent.) Browne next employs his senses, and cannot detect the difference himself, even though the country people give him a clue: 'the brevity by most imputed unto the left,' he repeats. This is the extent of his visual inspection. He never does the obvious thing of pointing us in the direction of a skeleton we might measure – that is what any dusty scholar would do. What he really wishes to do is get us to use our powers of God-given reason. Look at the 'total set of Animals' he instructs: their legs are always the same length on each side. For the badger to be different would simply be 'repugnant unto the course of Nature'. I am reluctant to settle for this theoretical rationale. It seems uncharacteristically dry. I have a vision of Browne offering more persuasive evidence, perhaps telling how he tethered a badger to a tree and then induced it to circulate in either direction in order to see if it ran better in one or the other.

Another time, I am watching the artist Marcus Coates entering one of his trance-like states in which he claims to speak with animal spirits. He is wearing a badger pelt, and in empathizing with his performance I involuntarily imagine myself doing the same. It takes this imagined substitution to remind me that I have one leg shorter than the other – and in fact the left – a minor deformity unnoticed by doctors and PE teachers, and by me, until in adulthood I learnt to ski and found that I could turn left more smoothly than right because of the difficulty in planting my short leg down the slope.

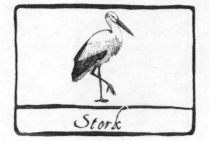

Stork

In 1668, a stork – a rare bird in these isles – is shot on the Norfolk coast near Happisburgh. It is brought to Browne alive with only its wing damaged. He feeds it on snails and frogs, and notes the clattering noise it makes when it snaps its bill together. He draws pictures of it to send to his daughter Elizabeth. Its feet have human-like nails rather than claws, 'such as Herodotus describeth the white Ibis of Ægypt to have'.

Browne is amused when visitors comment on his acquisition and repeat the superstition that storks prosper only in republics; hopefully, the bird does not foretoken a new commonwealth, they joke. He has already dispatched this error in *Pseudodoxia Epidemica*, written during England's own experiment with republicanism, the Commonwealth under Oliver Cromwell. Offering a rare clue to his political sympathies, Browne dismisses the republican stork as no more than 'a petty conceit to advance the opinion of popular policies'. For good measure, he adds a list of monarchies from ancient Egypt and Thessalia to modern France and Turkey where the bird nests without apparent regard to the system of governance. The Happisburgh stork arrives eight years after the Restoration of the monarchy, and Browne's satisfaction at the settled national state of affairs is palpable in his letters. With such a reputation hanging round its neck, it is easy to see why a stork arriving on the Norfolk coast, perhaps having flown in from the Dutch Republic, might be shot on sight.

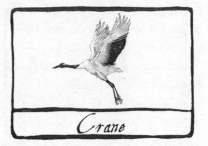

Crane

Browne's list of birds displays a preponderance of long-legged waders, reflecting his interest in helping Merret by ensuring that he includes in his natural history these typical residents of Norfolk's wetlands that he may not be aware of. Among these species, the largest and most extravagant is the common crane, with its couture smoke-grey plumage, black and white neck and blood-red highlight above the eye. 'Cranes are often seen here in hard winters especially about the champian & Feildie part it seems they have been more plentifull for in a bill of fare when the maior entertaind the duke of norfolk I meet with Cranes in a dish.' For this reason, and owing to systematic drainage of the land, the birds quickly became less plentiful and had died out in Norfolk by the end of the seventeenth century.

Today, they are making a cautious return, and a pair or more has bred successfully every year since 1982. More birds join these residents each winter, probably from Scandinavia. For a while, their preferred location was kept secret, but it is hard to keep secret a bird with a wingspan of over two metres that struts about as if auditioning for *Strictly Come Dancing*. Entirely by chance one day, I see a small flock of them in a winter field of beet tops, fanned out like a police forensic team combing the land for evidence or a body, each picking assiduously from the ground with its massive bill, its rump lifting with the action, allowing its tail feathers to wave in the breeze. There are about fifteen birds, surely enough to comprise a sedge, which is the approved collective noun for a group of cranes. The word has nothing to do with the riverside vegetation of that name. Nor is it, I think, simply an alternative spelling of siege, a military term that applies well to herons, which wait motionless for hours until their prey is forced from cover, but not to the foraging cranes. In Browne's time a sedge was also a formal assembly of noblemen, and given their stylish appearance and self-important attitudinizing, I feel this is the meaning that best fits these birds.

Cranes are 'the epitome of wild places,' according to the naturalist Richard Mabey. Perhaps he has in mind their saurian trumpeting call that can be heard for miles. For the landscape in which I see them is hardly wild. The crane was once a common bird in Britain. Although it is all but absent now, its spirit lives on in up to 300 English place names, such as Cranfield and Cranbrook, more than for any other bird, even the crow. Norfolk contributes a Cranwich and a Cranworth. The crane has much going for it as a focal species for conservation efforts. It is large, beautiful and entertaining. It pulls off the dual miracle of not only seeming exotic, but also of endeavouring to return to places it once called home. Like the kite, it is given a warmer welcome because it was us who first drove it away.

What is this bestiary, this list of animals imagined and real, seen by Browne, seen by me? What meaning should I extract from these fragmentary stories?

The set of real animals and the set of fictional animals do not of course overlap – nothing can be both real and fictional – but nor do they quite form a totality. In between lie other sets: creatures that have gone extinct and that now exist only in memory and as relics and fragments; creatures so rare that most people know nothing of them; and creatures not yet discovered.

Browne can rattle off a list of the notable birds and fishes of Norfolk, but he has no concept of which species might be 'endangered'. He is clear, though, on the principle of preventing harm. He regrets the prospect of an animal going extinct at man's hand: 'it was a vain design, that is, to destroy any species, or mutilate the great accomplishment of six days [i.e. the biblical creation]'. Surprisingly, he does not discuss the dodo, although his Norfolk friend Hamon l'Estrange at Hunstanton saw one in London in 1638. The bird was discovered only in 1598, the last specimen sighted in 1662; by 1681, it was extinct. The last aurochs, a species of wild cattle, was seen in Poland in 1627. The wolf disappeared from the British Isles during Browne's lifetime. The age of anthropogenic extinctions was hitting its stride. Because they haven't seen wolves within memory, Browne finds that 'common people have proceeded into opinions, and some wise men into affirmations' that the animals are incapable of living in Britain at all. How long does an animal have to be unfamiliar, or fully extinct, before we forget its true niche in nature? Not long, it seems. How long before its only habitat is the tapestry or the printed page where it becomes fabulous?

During ten years or more living in Norfolk, I have observed many variations in animal populations, but I have a hard time making sense of them. I see fewer swallows. I no longer hear the turtle doves that I was delighted to find purring in my garden when I first came here. But there are more buzzards and more Egyptian geese. Little egrets, a now frequent sight on the coast and on inland streams in the winter, were never listed even among the vagrant species in my childhood bird books. They are now well established in much of England, having worked their way steadily northward since their first landfall in Dorset in 1989, a bellwether of cleaner waters or of a warming climate.

I read that there is a thousand-fold increase in the rate of animal extinction above the natural level, owing to man's hunting, land clearance, urbanization and pollution. This ongoing loss is mostly met, if not with outright apathy, then with despairing resignation. In the space of a few decades, the tense and mood of the discussion have slipped from the present imperative to the past indifferent. A tone of lament is now routine in nature writing, not only in polemical works aiming to draw our attention to the dangers of species loss, but from almost any writer who finds himself or herself out in (more or less) wild surroundings. It is as if this were enough. A proposal called the Memo Project goes a stage further, planning the erection of a 'beautiful monument to species going extinct worldwide' on the Isle of Portland, with a bell that will ring for each new extinction. (Memo stands for Mass Extinction Monitoring Observatory.) The intended Donnean message to humanity is clear enough ('...It tolls for thee'), but I find something obscene about this ostentatious mourning too soon substituted for effective remedial action. In writing that I 'no longer' hear turtle doves, I realize I have unwittingly joined this lament. In truth, I do not know if 'no longer' is the right phrase. The birds have missed several summers (some of them eminently missable), but I suppose they may always return next year. I hope so.

An objective measure of changing biodiversity is hard to achieve. Our scientific censuses and methods of estimating numbers are fairly recent. Before that, we have only the sporadic diaries of naturalists and anecdotal sightings to go by. The recorded loss of an individual species makes for a neat tragic episode, but the pattern of overall losses is both harder to gauge and harder to make into a satisfactory story. Yet with the inability to sense the pattern comes the capacity to deny it. Today, we are in the paradoxical position of knowing that many creatures are going extinct before they have even enjoyed the dubious privilege of being discovered by man. Occasionally, a spectacular new animal is found. In 2013, it was not a unicorn but the olinguito, an arboreal mammal from the forests of Ecuador and Colombia, that was identified by naturalists from the Smithsonian Institution. Although it eats fruit, the olinguito is also carnivorous and so it was classified among the *Carnivora*, which includes cats and bears, which instantly made it seem a more striking find – the first addition to that order of mammals for more than thirty years. We do not yet know which species went extinct during that year. It may be some creature we never knew.

In Browne's time, many animals were only known by unreliable verbal reports and artists' illustrations, whereas now we can observe the intimate lives of obscure species on television. At the same time, we are more physically disconnected from nature than ever, and are maintained in a more subtle kind of ignorance. Nature programmes tell us how to think about animals, but the instruction they give may be no less biased and self-serving than the fables of old. According to Brett Mills, who researches popular television at the University of East Anglia, they may even be a surreptitious means of promulgating normative models of *human* behaviour. The narration is carefully constructed, pronounced either by an unseen 'voice of God', or by a trusted presenter speaking in hushed and reverent tones to camera (evoking thoughts respectively of Eden and church). Camera shots are framed to emphasize the wildness of the environment, carefully excluding the paraphernalia of the film crew and other evidence of human disturbance, tacitly acknowledging that one role of these films is to answer our vicarious lust for wilderness. The overall effect is to deliver an intensity of aesthetic experience quite unlike that to be found in the authentic environment. The action-packed hour of a typical nature programme is an hour that I know I could spend observing a single heron standing motionless on the bank of a stream waiting for prey.

High-definition images tell a low-definition story. The focus is usually on the life and habits of a single species, often a single member of that species. Sometimes, it has even been given a human name. All of this belies the complexity of species interaction and interdependence that is the binding thread in the story of life on earth. The conventions of the narrative arc require certain things to happen within the edited hour: we know that the famously elusive animal will appear eventually, we know we will see the predator catch the prey, but not before we have also seen the prey make a 'lucky' escape. There are other tropes, too: the annual migration that is treated as an epic journey; the fight for the fittest to mate and survive; the mutually sustaining relationship that reflects our own ideal of society. When Mills compared the story lines of nature documentaries with accounts of the same animals' lives in the zoology literature, he also found a disproportionate emphasis on heterosexuality, monogamy and good parenting. Who does not now know about the male penguin that looks after the pair's lone egg? What a fine role model he is for modern fatherhood. Meanwhile, behaviours that are unacceptable in humans, but that may be perfectly natural in the species under the camera, such as autophagy (eating parts of one's own body, seen for example in octopuses) and cannibalism (eating others of the same species), are screened in the interests of scientific honesty but accompanied by expressions of appropriate distaste.

The very landscape in which these animals perform their antics has also probably been subject to manipulation. In most places, there is no truly 'natural' environment left, only a choice between varieties of human ideas of the natural. Take your pick of our agricultural landscape (England's green and pleasant land to some, but 'sheep-wrecked', in George Monbiot's word, and reduced to a sterile monoculture), or the intensively managed wetlands of the RSPB, which are from time to time relocated in order to 'protect' them, ironically, against natural events such as coastal floods. In his manifesto for 'rewilding' the countryside, Monbiot gives unwitting expression to the paradox we face, when he writes with unconscious hubris of 'allowing' nature to find its own way towards his chosen utopia. As nature is from time to time apt to remind us, it does not need our permission.

These are our contemporary delusions. The 'pathetic fallacy' of the sentimental poets who ascribed human emotions to animals that John Ruskin sought to skewer in 1856 has been extended to a shameless anthropomorphism in almost all mediated presentations of the animal kingdom, from cartoon feature films to supposedly scientific documentaries. In place of the symbolic representation of animals in the emblems of Browne's day, we now have animals projected back to us as models of human behaviour. The dolphin was once emblematic of speed or haste, often depicted in conjunction with an anchor, 'implying that common moral, Festina lente', as Browne explains. Now, though, it is our aquatic doppelgänger, an icon of animal intelligence, dominant in its environment, but also innocent and playful, like Man before the Fall. Both images are false.

What hope is there for 'rewilding' ourselves if we cannot even see these creatures accurately for what they are in the wild – in their wild?

And what hope is there that we will learn to regard animals neither as objects nor as quasi-persons, but as animals, animals in an ecosystem that we share? 'The world was made to be inhabited by beasts,' Browne wrote, 'but studied and contemplated by man: 'tis the debt of our reason wee owe unto God, and the homage wee pay for not being beasts.'

4

Plants

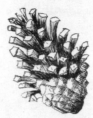

'inexcusable Pythagorisme'
The Garden of Cyrus

VISITING THOMAS BROWNE in 1671, the diarist John Evelyn called 'his whole house and garden…a paradise and cabinet of rarities, and that of the best collection, especially medals, books, plants, and natural things'. Praise indeed from the renowned author of *Sylva*, a 'Discourse of Forest Trees', translator of French gardening manuals, and author of the first book on salad plants.

The exact boundaries of this town garden are not known. Taking Evelyn's fulsome description at face value, the garden and the house appear as a contiguous intellectual space, with plants as curious and varied as the precious objects and books indoors. Whatever its extent, it was not enough for Browne's purposes, as he later leased a small meadow from the Dean and Chapter of Norwich Cathedral.

What did he grow? The keeping of a garden for the pleasure of its flowers was brought to Norwich by the Dutch. The city held Florists' Feasts and Browne noted the faddism of the 'tulipists'. More important for a physician was the growing of medicinal plants. During his studies in Montpellier and Padua, Browne had the opportunity to explore the first botanic gardens, the models for later gardens in Oxford and Paris, at

Kew, and elsewhere, which all set out with the principal aim of growing and studying plants that might have medical therapeutic effects.

The Chelsea Physic Garden in London, founded in 1673 by the Worshipful Company of Apothecaries, is the garden that is today clearest about these origins, in title at least. I enter through a gateway in a high brick wall overhung with climbing hydrangea, and am immediately disappointed to find that its pharmaceutical garden is not a seventeenth-century replica, but is laid out according to modern medical disciplines – cardiology, gastroenterology and so on. Many of the plants are the ones Browne knew, though. The 'Anaesthesia and analgesia' section, for instance, has *Mandragora officinarum*, the mandrake which was once believed to shriek when pulled from the ground, and whose stout root often bifurcates so that it resembles the figure of a man (especially when a small third rootstalk is present). An active substance in this root, I read on the label, is now made synthetically for use in preoperative anaesthesia. Belladonna, digitalis and the opium poppy are among the plants I find in 'cardiology'. Liquorice, traditionally used

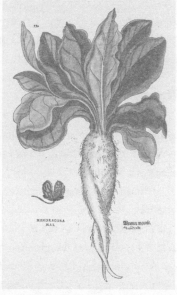

in the treatment of indigestion, has recently been found effective in reducing stomach ulcers. It is favoured as a natural remedy and chemists have derived a synthetic drug from it. Pellitory-of-the-wall, a member of the *Urticaceae* family, was a remedy for a dry cough, short breath and wheezing. Asparagus was prescribed to stir up lust. It reminds me that the appearance of plants was often taken as a clue to their medical application. Who's to say this seventeenth-century Viagra doesn't work even today, innuendo being perhaps as effective as pharmacology? Asparagus still makes regular appearances on lists of supposed aphrodisiac foods.

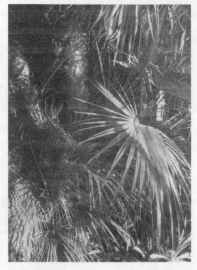

The botanical garden in Padua, established in 1545, still contains a few of the very same plants that Browne saw growing, notable among them the so-called 'Goethe palm', said to be the tree that prompted the German author to write his *Metamorphosis of Plants*. It had been growing for two centuries when Goethe saw it, and so Browne, too, had surely observed how each leaf, forming as a single blade low down, splits along fine longitudinal creases as it grows and spreads into feathery fronds higher up the tree. Padua's beds of medicinal plants are more comprehensive than Chelsea's, and they are less worried about alerting visitors to the poisonous species. A ricin plant, a species often considered as a biological warfare agent, blossoms with comical crimson pompoms at head height. A fruiting red chilli is described as 'rubefacente' – restoring redness to the skin – another medicinal prescription based on visual suggestion.

Browne's own garden surely supplied him with a few of these plants, although as a modern physician he perhaps relied more on apothecaries to make up his preparations. It meant more to him though as a place of contemplation, wonder and enquiry, somewhere that he could observe the ever-changing patterns made by nature. The meadow near Pull's Ferry on the River Wensum served a more extreme version of this purpose. It was a kind of experiment allowed to run out of control, an early example of Monbiotian 'rewilding', as he seems to have let it go simply for the pleasure of seeing what would grow there without cultivation.

Browne's list of Norfolk birds and fishes was the workmanlike product of a specific request from a fellow scholar. But his botanical work soon opens out into something far more ambitious. This encyclopedia of Norfolk plants – for it is almost entirely from indigenous plants that he draws his inspiration – bears the daunting title *The Garden of Cyrus, or the Quincunciall, Lozenge, or Network Plantations of the Ancients, Artificially, Naturally, Mystically Considered*. The text is abundant and rhapsodic, even apparently chaotic. But, concerned as it is with patterns of order in nature, it is itself deeply ordered. It purports to be about the ancient Persian custom of planting orchards in a particular design, but Browne quickly abstracts from this idea the geometric form of the quincunx, the X shape made by five points arranged as on the face of a die, and from that launches into a broader exploration of the occurrence and significance of the number five in nature.

This is no work of obscure numerology as you might expect, but one that hovers tantalizingly on the verge of true scientific revelation.

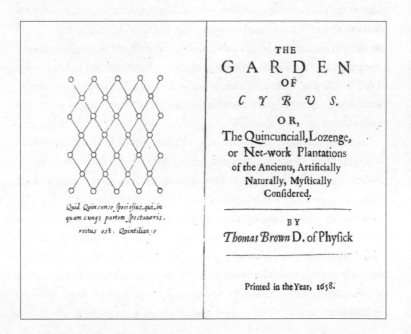

Quid Quincunce speciosius, qui, in
quam cunq; partem spectaueris,
rectus est. Quintilian: 9

THE
GARDEN
OF
C Y R U S.
OR,
The Quincunciall, Lozenge,
or Net-work Plantations
of the Ancients, Artificially
Naturally, Mystically
Considered.

BY
Thomas Brown D. of Physick

Printed in the Year, 1658.

The essay unfolds almost literally like a flower, for four short chapters, dealing with this geometry and matters arising from it may be peeled back, as it were, from the long central chapter, the 'naturally considered' portion, which holds the essential content, the seed head of the work, a roll call of plants observed by Browne to exhibit a five-fold patterning. While it is the outer chapters that have delighted and puzzled literary admirers, with their bravura displays of Browne's mature style, it is this central chapter that contains the kernel of science.

I myself hate gardens. Or, to be more exact, I hate the duties of a garden; I hate garden*ing*. I can luxuriate in a garden that others have gone to the trouble of creating, and am happy to admire its maker's talent and skill, and the richness and variety of plant forms that have erupted, consequently or not, from their actions.

But few things dismay me more than my own garden. The very sight of it reproaches me with chores undone. Just an hour of struggling to clear a bed of nettles is enough for me. I can never clear my head of the obvious futility of the task. I rage against the tangle of roots and the stinging. How can it be that so many plants in an English garden scratch and sting? My aversion is partly owing to the fact that the burden of my task is to do with killing – trimming bushes, cutting down dying trees, mowing what we laughingly call the lawn (it is mostly moss, and if it were entirely so, that would be fine by me). I tell myself that this work is essential too, all part of the natural cycle, but it does no good.

There is a deeper annoyance. I have a theory that gardens are a project for people who have given up on intellectual commerce and ideas. The garden is for them what it is so often said to be, a refuge and a solace. Plants may not conform exactly to one's will, but they may be nurtured or rooted out, and led towards a certain destiny. Our ideas for them determine their prospects – something we cannot enforce in the case of people. It is strange to me that gardeners' refuge from the chaos of human interaction should be a riot of nature, a mirroring chaos of growth and mindless competition to match the human rat race.

How did Browne feel about gardens? He tells us rather little about this in *The Garden of Cyrus*. It is notable that many of the plants he describes are those that were, and in many cases still are, to be found in any field or hedgerow. Perhaps he preferred to pass time in his wild meadow than in his tidy physic garden. I would certainly prefer to pass the time in Browne's meadow. Sadly, I cannot. After Browne died, the land was used as a vegetable garden for the cathedral, then as allotments for residents in the Cathedral Close, until the 1970s, when it was turned into a private car park.

The garden can be a space for philosophy. Limbo, the first circle of hell described in *Inferno*, is a garden ringed by seven castle walls. Its denizens, Dante tells us, are men of worth, who are not sinners but who, by accident of chronology or geography, have never had the opportunity of baptism. They include Browne's principal classical sources, not only the philosophers Heraclitus, Empedocles, Socrates, Plato and Aristotle, but also the physicians Galen, Avicenna, and Averroës.

Yet the garden itself and the activity of gardening have, like many

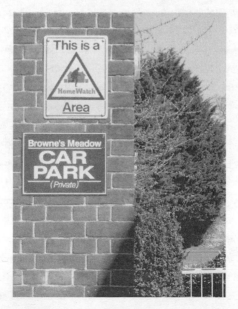

popular pastimes, received rather little philosophical attention. Francis Bacon in his *Essays* of 1625 called gardens 'the purest of human pleasures'. In a period when sex and even food carried the taint of sin, this is a perhaps expected observation. I am sure many people still believe this, without even taking an ironic pause to note how much this purity is based on the display of plants' sexual parts. Bacon went on to divulge his rational plan for a garden, basically comprising a hedged square of lawn, the most conventional view of the garden as a symbol of man's control over nature, and an ideal that still dominates the suburban English imagination.

For many, it is enough that gardens give pleasure, without asking what it is that constitutes the pleasure. Some say a garden is a means of better appreciating nature. But this is not it: the way to appreciate nature must be to get out into nature itself. Others refine this idea. For Bacon, the garden is the 'first ornamentall Scene of nature'. This is better. But who decides what is ornamental and what is not? Most philosophers of the garden do not really tackle this essential aspect of artifice, the fact that it matters that what one nurtures and trains ultimately *looks* as if it has been nurtured and trained, at least a little bit. The goal of some of the most admired gardens (Japanese gardens, or the temporary creations of the Chelsea Flower Show, for example) seems to be to improve on nature, to bring it to a state of perfection, but in order to do this they must practically exclude nature altogether. For others, a 'wild' garden is more desirable, but this of course may require just as much artful arrangement. In both cases, it is nature and artifice brought together in chosen proportions that matters. The constant tension between these two, between the intention of man and the latent potential for nature to take its independent course (either bringing to full expression man's intention or gradually, picturesquely, demolishing it), is what distinguishes the garden from the truly wild.

Like Bacon, Browne loves a garden for its own sake as well as for its useful plants. But he is not persuaded by the rigours of the Baconian design. Browne lived before Western civilization developed its sentimental idea of nature as an aesthetic resource. Our concepts of landscape and wilderness were not articulated until the eighteenth century; they would have meant very little to him. Yet he appreciates chaos and chance, the bramble strangling the clipped beech hedge, the blown rose as well as the perfect bud. Again, we find Browne far ahead of the fashion.

He would have enjoyed other things, too. It is notable in the philosophical discussion of gardens today that the actual plants in them seem to play little or no part. The meaning of gardens seems to exist entirely separately from the meanings once ascribed to individual plants. For Browne, almost every plant had a medicinal purpose or an emblematic association. The garden was then a kind of library, a place of half-remembered stories. This allusive, even allegorical, aspect of the garden is now a closed book to most of us.

Apart from pretty flowers and the utilitarian satisfaction of growing plants for food (and, in Browne's case, medicine), what else do we have? What about the activity itself? According to David Cooper, writing in *A Philosophy of Gardens*: 'It is symptomatic of a primarily aesthetic approach largely to ignore the practice of gardening.' Yet there is a benefit to physical health – if all that fresh air can be said to outweigh the effect on the knees and back. And there is a purported benefit to mental health. A spell of 'gardening leave' – the genteel euphemism favoured by the British Civil Service when an employee is laid off – has connotations of a sabbatical or nature cure. There is even a charity called Gardening Leave set up to help military veterans with mental health issues through horticultural therapy. A recent piece of research by psychologists at the University of Munich – widely cited by authors of self-help books, though less so by other scientists – even suggests that brief glimpses of the colour green are enough to trigger greater human creativity. The words 'green' and 'grow' are etymologically linked, according to the paper's author, Stephanie Lichtenfeld. The meaning we attach to the colour may stretch 'from the concrete notion of vegetative growth and life to the more abstract, psychological notions of development and mastery'. Rory Stuart finds more spiritual answers in his book *What Are Gardens For?* He believes gardening inculcates virtues of care, self-discipline and humility (a word that derives, as he points out, from the Latin *humus*, meaning earth). 'We gardeners,' he writes, 'feel the tranquillity of being among living things that do not move and make little noise, that obey a cyclical rhythm that is not our own, and over which we have limited influence.'

I understand in an obscure way that all these virtues – even the mutually contradictory ones of taking care and letting go – are present in the activity of gardening. I well up without fail at the end of *Candide*, when Candide and Cunégonde sing the final number, 'Make Our Garden Grow'. Is this emotional release entirely an effect of the music, or do the words have something to do with it? I feel all of a sudden that keeping a garden is a profoundly moral thing to do. In the original Voltaire, the line is: 'Il faut cultiver notre jardin.' It is a metaphorical as well as horticultural envoi: we should stick to our knitting, we should keep calm and carry on, because there's always work to do in a garden.

But then my unease returns, because being asked simply to 'carry on' immediately prompts the rejoinder: 'What's the alternative?' I am reminded of the opening lines of the monologue in Samuel Beckett's novel *The Unnamable*: 'Keep going, going on. Call that going? Call that on?' I am back where I started. I'm with Franz Kafka, from whose diary Beckett pulled out this dyspeptic quote: 'Gardening. No hope for the future.'

Browne's near-contemporary Andrew Marvell was preoccupied with the meaning of gardens, and wrote many poems on the subject. In 'The Garden', he is savage about our tendency to congratulate ourselves on growing what nature might grow anyway without our help:

> How vainly men themselves amaze
> To win the palm, the oak, or bays,
> And their uncessant labours see
> Crown'd from some single herb or tree.

Though Browne admires Cyrus (the Younger, a prince of Persia in the fifth century BCE) as 'Not only a Lord of Gardens, but a manuall planter thereof', it is doubtful that he did much spadework himself. He sought out rare seeds and made careful notes of where they were planted and whether they came up, but he still considers that he 'was never the master of any considerable garden'. Nor I.

Perhaps I can overcome my aversion and even find illumination if I plant a garden for myself. I will make a square bed. In the autumn, I will plant four trees in the corners and one in the centre to make a quincunx. Now, though, it is spring, and I will seek out some of the smaller plants that Browne celebrates in *The Garden of Cyrus*. Many I find growing – by accident or by design – in my garden already. The walnut, hazel and alder all have catkins that display the lozenge patterning that Browne describes. The sycamore and the fig have new palmate leaves made up of five fingers. Later in the year I will see the 'squamous heads' of scabious and knapweed, artichoke and teasel. Always there high on the wall if I need a quincunxial reference point are clusters of *Sempervivum*, '*Jupiters* beard, or houseleek; which old superstitions set on the tops of houses, as a defensative against lightening'. I know from personal experience that the plant is no defence against lightning, but I can see that its tight rosettes of succulent leaves do provide durable evidence of the occurrence of the number five in plants. I twist one away from the wall and label the leaves in sequence as they spiral out from the centre. When I have done, I have five distinct whorls, and every leaf is accounted for.

I scan seed catalogues searching for some of the rarer plants Browne names, but find few matches. Perhaps his examples are now considered to be weeds, or have become unfashionable, or else the names have changed over the years. I am especially disappointed not to be able to track down the 'man *Orchis* of *Columna*', an orchid whose flower has no five-fold property but the shape of a man – 'well made out, it excelleth in all analogies,' says Browne. Eventually, I order seeds of salsify and asphodel, the flower said to carpet the meadows of the underworld.

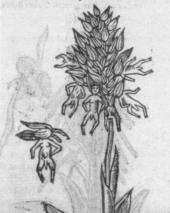

Orchis Anthropophora Oreades mas.
The male Neapolitan Fooleſtones.

Then I select a neglected patch of turf and begin to clear a square of earth in readiness.

'Gardens were before Gardiners, and but some hours after the earth,' Browne concludes in the opening paragraph of *The Garden of Cyrus*. It's a slick phrase, another quotable quote. What does he really mean? In the first book of Genesis, God creates the plant kingdom – grass and the herb yielding seed and the tree yielding fruit – three days before he introduces man. This is how there can be a garden before gardeners, although Genesis 2 immediately contradicts this version by implying that it needed both rain and man to till the ground before Eden could be made.

A garden is not just grass and herbs and trees, however. It must also display evidence of artful arrangement. The garden of the third day, then, must have God's design upon it, which means that each and every plant carries within it evidence of God's creation.

Browne approaches the plants of Norfolk quite differently from the way he considers its animals. The animals are curiosities, to be described and listed, foolish misunderstandings about them to be cleared up as he goes. The plants warrant deeper enquiry. It is as if they hold the key to something. Browne of course already has every reason to believe that they do, as so many of them are the basis of medical cures. While delighting in his powers of scientific observation, he hopes to discern signs of the original garden, Eden, amid the chaotic undergrowth of East Anglia.

In doing this, he anticipates his own desired sight of Paradise. For Browne, the aspects of gardening that we tend to gloss over – the cutting back, the rotting vegetation – are to be celebrated as much as any blossom.

The autumn of decay and dying is the prelude to nature's regeneration in the shoots of spring and to man's own resurrection. The garden is a lifelong place of religious inspiration. Through study of its regenerative powers, he writes in *Religio Medici*: 'no true Scholler becomes an Atheist, but from the visible effects of nature, growes up a reall Divine'.

Our lives are spent distinguishing between order and disorder. We are adapted to recognize order in nature because a disruption of that order may be key to our survival – it may indicate prey moving through the long grass or fruit hidden among the leaves. We discern visual order when the repetition of similar units (blades of grass, leaves) forms an array or pattern. The essential components of a pattern are space and number. The interplay of these two factors is formally described by the language of symmetry (the mirror symmetry of a face, the rotational symmetry of many flowers, the translational symmetry of a row of vines, say).

According to Browne, 'nature Geometrizeth, and observeth order in all things'. For him, order in nature is a clue to the ways of the innocent world before the Fall, and patterns of growth and repetition are auguries of renewal, rebirth and resurrection. (Order is an ambiguous word, of course, encompassing social and moral order as well as visual order in nature, a thought that cannot be far from Browne's mind, writing *The Garden of Cyrus* during the later years of Cromwell's Protectorate.)

Number is an index of this natural order. 'I have often admired the mysticall way of *Pythagoras*, and the secret magicke of numbers,' Browne writes. But he is no numerologist who believes that certain numbers have significance in themselves. He follows a number if it leads somewhere, but not beyond the point of reason. When he explores the supposed significance of man's 'climactericall', or sixty-third, year, he is led naturally to that number's factors, seven and nine, and from there notes the traditional division of human life into seven-year stages of maturity, for example. But he is careful to add the sceptical note that at one time or another 'all or most' numbers have been 'mystically applauded'. He cites one, for the unity of God; three, for the mystery of the Trinity; four, the

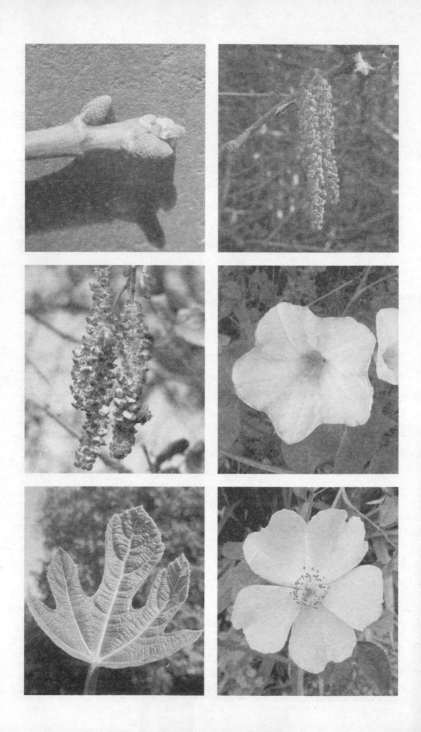

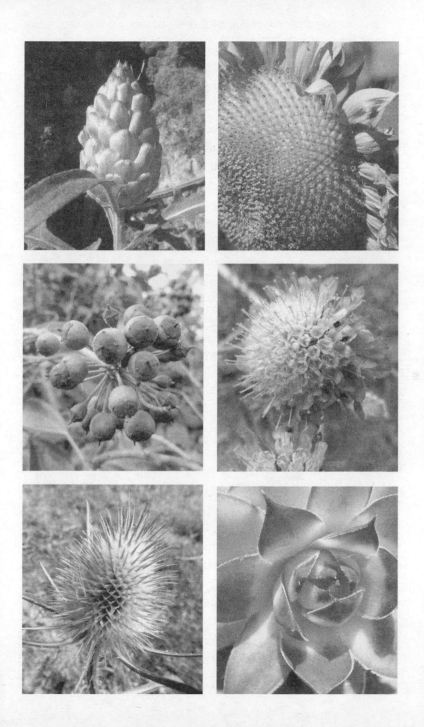

number of the elements as well as the number of letters in the name of God in Hebrew and various other ancient languages; six, which is a perfect number (its factors add up to itself) as well as the number of days of the creation; and ten, which we use as our number base for counting.

It is notable that Browne's reasons for the significance of these numbers are drawn from human culture. If he had included nature in his argument, he would have been able to add the missing numbers, the two of bilateral animals, the eight of the octopus and spider, and above all the five of the starfish and so many flowers.

Yet in *The Garden of Cyrus*, paradoxically, Browne's gallery of specimen plants doesn't really serve his ostensible rhetorical purpose of persuading us that the number five is special. It leaves us instead with the delicious feeling that he could just as easily have done the same for any number. The work is a vehicle for Browne's typical genius of weaving an entertaining distraction from any 'bye and barren Theme'.

This casualness is all the more tantalizing because we know now that the number five really is a key to the secret of natural growth. In 1202, the mathematician Leonardo of Pisa, known as Fibonacci, published a book of number puzzles called *Liber Abaci*, which included one conundrum about rabbit-breeding. The problem was this: starting with one pair of rabbits, how many pairs will you have after so many generations? Conveniently, the rabbits live for ever, and breed when they are exactly a month old and monthly after that, producing a pair of male and female young each time. The number of pairs each month is given by the sequence that now bears Fibonacci's name, in which each number is the sum of the two immediately preceding numbers: 1, 1, 2, 3, 5, 8, 13, 21, 34, 55 and so on. As the series advances, the ratio of adjacent terms (1:1, 2:1, 3:2, 5:3, etc.) approaches the proportion known as the golden ratio: 1.618034…Both the numbers of the sequence and the forms that can be constructed based on the golden ratio are abundant in nature.

Fortunately, the numbers of the sequence often emerge in natural patterns that don't bounce around as much as rabbits. They surface, for example, in the angular spacing between successive leaves on a stem, the constant angle being one of the fractions of a circle given by the Fibonacci sequence: one half, one third, one fifth, and so on. They appear more obviously in the tighter arrays of pine-cone scales and clustered florets of composite flowers, where adjacent numbers in the series govern the way they spiral out from the centre where they are formed (and where the biological process of cell division takes the place of replicating rabbits as the generating process behind the numbers). I saw five spirals of leaves in my *Sempervivum*. Returning to my cutting, I find that these run anticlockwise out from the centre of the rosette. Looking closely, I now see that there is a second, steeper set of spirals running clockwise. I count them; there are eight, the number after five in the sequence.

The systematic investigation of these arrangements did not really get going until the nineteenth century, when it was named phyllotaxis (from the Greek words for leaf and arrangement). The revelation that the plant kingdom contained a hidden law of numbers prompted works of wonder, such as John Hutton Balfour's *Botany and Religion, or Illustrations of the Works of God in the Structure, Functions, Arrangement, and General Distribution of Plants* of 1859, but scientists were left puzzled as to how this could aid their efforts to understand botanical structures. It turns out that it is in fact possible to classify every plant species in terms of two adjacent numbers of the Fibonacci sequence. Many plants display this underlying mathematics in the disposition of leaves around their stems, or more obviously in flower petals and seed heads. But there is more. Scientists have recently found that it is possible to produce the same spiral patterns in entirely *physical* systems, for example when magnetic droplets take up positions in a suitable magnetic field. The Fibonacci sequence turns out to be not the exclusive property of biology but something linked to fundamental physical laws. Yet it seems that this exciting empirical observation still awaits the theory that will fully explain it.

Throughout his catalogue of plants, Browne seems to be on the verge of discerning the Fibonacci sequence. But he is not a mathematician and nowhere uses mathematics to assist his argument, as Descartes was able to do in his description of the logarithmic spiral, or as the architect Inigo Jones did in his design for the beautiful spiral staircase of the Queen's House, Greenwich, both of which rely on the golden ratio.

And Browne is, besides, fatally distracted from this course by the lure of the quincunx.

At the end of May, the first frail tendrils of salsify appear in the modules I have seeded. It is supposedly one of those moments when the pleasure of gardening is made manifest. You are given something back for your efforts, a reward, a new creation. I am moderately pleased, but more frustrated at the complete non-appearance of my asphodels. Plants either grow or they do not. In truth, I feel I have had little to do with their progress. My greatest happiness so far has come from preparing a perfect bare square of earth.

Now it is time to plant out. I have bought some asphodelines to replace the failed asphodels, and a species of sunflower. The sun is hot and it is almost still. I quickly develop a sweat as I dig holes for them. I find the tools less than ideal for the task and end up scooping earth with cupped hands. None of it is a joy. I bed the plants in and water them. A few days later I check on them. They seem to have taken well, but my main satisfaction is to see that my square is still free of weeds.

From time to time through the summer I monitor progress. The sunflowers bloom, and I count their petals. Each flower has thirteen petals – another Fibonacci number – and their seed heads radiate in thirteen nested arcs. One morning in September, I find that although the bees are enjoying the sunflowers, deer have also been enjoying my salsify. They have chewed off all the tops in the night and now I must re-bed the disturbed roots and hope they regenerate.

My efforts in the garden are less dogged than those of Gustave Flaubert's *Bouvard and Pécuchet*, but I notice that my reactions are similar. Like them, I find myself exclaiming at what has grown: 'They took pleasure in naming aloud all the vegetables: "Look, carrots! Ah, cabbages!"' This is the conventional response to the 'miracle' of growth, or, more particularly, to the miracle that (as we kid ourselves) we have grown these plants, our hubris there in the twisting of the verb into the transitive form.

Elsewhere in my garden, the number five is conspicuously recurrent. I have many of the plants that Browne lists as 'pentagonally wrapped up', from bindweed to roses, both wild ones with simple, five-petal flowers and fancy breeds, which have many more petals, but which, as Browne finds, still reveal their allegiance to the five-fold in their 'calicular leaves' or sepals. The five-fold seems special because it is odd, odd in both the phenomenal and the numeral sense. It lacks the more obvious natural symmetry that flowers with even numbers of petals have.

In *Timaeus*, Plato's description of the world, the philosopher aligns the four simplest Platonic solids, the tetrahedron, the cube, the octahedron and the icosahedron, with the four elements, fire, earth, air and water. The fifth and most complex solid, the pentagon-faced dodecahedron, represents the ether that suffuses the universe. It turns out that he wasn't far off the truth. Many molecules are built around pentagonal rings of bonded atoms, including my favourite, buckminsterfullerene. I found out that five-fold symmetry arises at many scales in nature. It is in the starfish and sea urchins that Thomas Browne knew, but also in the marine microorganisms known as radiolaria and in viruses that he did not know. It is perhaps even present at the atomic scale in the symmetry of the clouds of charge around atomic nuclei.

Five-fold symmetry was long thought to be absent from the mineral world of crystals because it is impossible to produce a space-filling array using repeating units based only on pentagonal geometry. Proper crystals are constrained to have two-, three-, four- or six-fold symmetry. However, in 1984, 'quasicrystals' with five-fold symmetry were observed in certain metal alloys, and many more have been discovered since. They have similarities with the tiling patterns mathematically described by Roger Penrose not long before, which incorporate star and pentagon tiles among other shapes to produce arrays that may be infinitely extended, but which, unlike a floor of square or hexagonal tiles, does

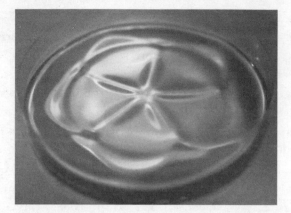

not incorporate periodic repetition. In 2013, physicists at the University of Nice even managed to produce standing waves based on stars and pentagons in vibrating pools of oil, something previously thought impossible. Browne might still exclaim today 'how nature delighteth in this number'.

Five-fold symmetry is mysteriously pervasive in human culture. It occurs as a decorative device on prehistoric pottery, and in Minoan and Mycenaean seals. It was a symbol first to the Pythagoreans, then to medieval astrologers and alchemists. It is associated with witchcraft: Goethe's Faust exorcises Mephistopheles using a pentagram (Goethe had also noted the prevalence of five-fold design in nature). Then there is the Pentagon itself, a building designed for the efficient circulation of staff, but which inevitably invites theories of more sinister symbolism. The design echoes the symmetry of earlier defensive structures, including many seventeenth-century forts, such as the Landguard Fort at Harwich, which Browne may have known.

The same symmetry is equally favoured on our own proletarian plane. A pentagon inscribed with a star forms the logo of the Chrysler car manufacturer, for example. Almost all modern office chairs possess five equally disposed feet. At what point was four no longer enough? Geoff Hollington, a friend who has designed such chairs, informs me that the change was prompted by safety regulations introduced in the 1970s with the aim of making it harder to fall over while sitting on chairs that now had the new hazard of castors on their feet. The geometry shows that one extra leg buys a considerable increase in the tipping force. But Geoff believes it is also a visual preference. 'Maybe we prefer this because it's familiarly what happens in nature.'

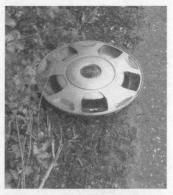

Another design commonplace, the car hubcap, supports this argument. These wheel covers obviously must have a basic circular symmetry. But they usually sport a decorative lower order of symmetry, too. Unlike chair legs, there is no mechanical reason to prefer five-fold symmetry, and yet this does seem to be the most common pattern.

The number five is equally pervasive in aural experience. The pentatonic scale – five notes so harmoniously spaced that they may form a pleasing tune no matter in what order they are played – forms the basis of folk music around the world. One work that makes conspicuous play of it is by the Japanese composer Tōru Takemitsu. His orchestral piece *A Flock Descends into the Pentagonal Garden*, composed in 1977, is based on a dream of his in which a flock of birds alights in the said garden, which turns out to be the curiously shaved head of the artist Marcel Duchamp as captured in a famous photograph by Man Ray.

'To enlarge this contemplation unto all the mysteries and secrets, accomodable unto this number, were inexcusable Pythagorisme,' writes Browne at the head of the fifth and final chapter of *The Garden of Cyrus*. He is showing some neck here, for he has already digressed far and wide, and now goes on to point out that five is the number of the senses and of the conic sections, and that, as it is written in Leviticus, the sinner who takes something that is not his must pay back one fifth extra above its value. For my part, I observe merely that VAT today stands at 20 per cent.

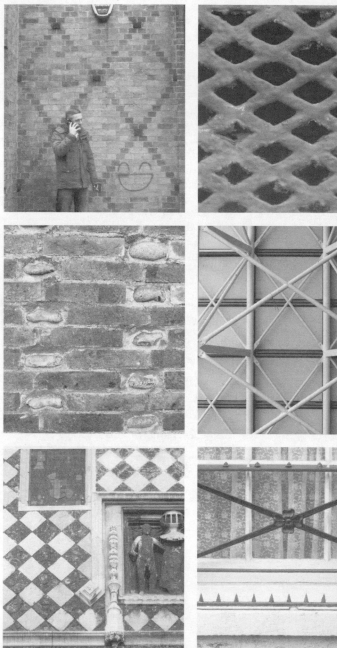

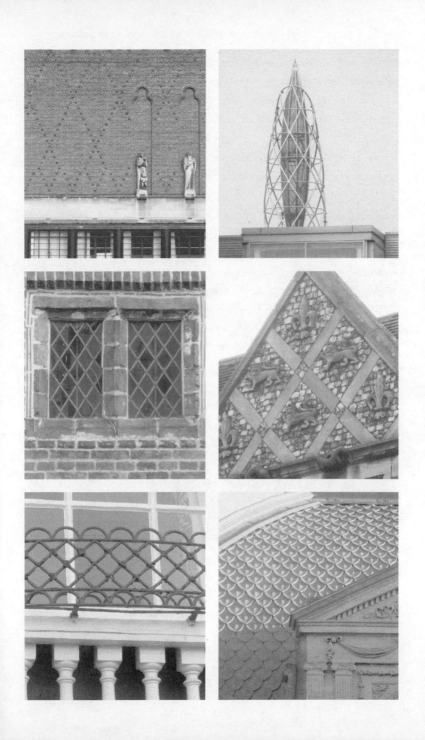

To anybody mathematically minded, the quincunx clearly has little to do with five-fold symmetry or the number five at all, although it turns out in the end, most surprisingly, that the gardeners of the 'network plantations of the ancients' and nature's phyllotaxis are chasing after the same goal.

Browne's quincunx is the diamond trellis he shows us in the frontis-piece of *The Garden of Cyrus*. It is a pattern seen, as he tells us, in catkins and pine cones and leaded windows and iron gratings and fishing nets. It is present singly in the X frame of Roman chair supports and in the way beds are lashed together. Above all, though, the quincunx is the template of the 'sacred Plantations of Antiquity', and perhaps even the Garden of Eden, which we know had at least the central tree of knowledge.

Quincunxes are out of fashion these days, but I find a grand remnant of some near Capel St Andrew in Suffolk along a straight mile or so of a road bordering the northern edge of Rendlesham Forest, a place haunted by Britain's most notorious UFO sighting. The trees are known as the

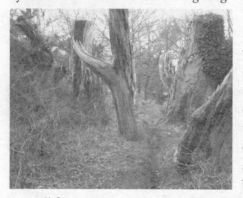

Butley Clumps. According-ing to one local story, they were planted in 1805 to celebrate Nelson's victory at Trafalgar, quintets chosen perhaps because of the year. All that remains of most of the quincunxes are one or two massive beech stumps, but in a few cases all four stumps survive, clearly disposed to the corners of a square, with a central trunk – this always a pine – also present. Here and there, an effort has been made to replant the missing clusters, with quadrates of sturdy beeches planted around their central Scots pines, all protected by rabbit-proof plastic mesh.

But the stumps are better. They have a memorial potency. I cannot tell how long ago the trees died or were felled, but they still serve as symbolic markers in the landscape. Walkers have worn a pathway along the verge of the road from quincunx to quincunx, passing through the middle of each, dodging round the central pine where necessary, threading them onto a continuous ley line.

Browne's diagram of a quincunx is in fact nothing more than the simplest of two-dimensional lattices. Its unit cell – the minimum module from which the array may be built and extended to infinity – is a square (or a rhombus, in Browne's elegant drawing). Each corner – the site of a tree in a quincunxial orchard – is equivalent. Each unit cell thus contains a quarter of a tree at each corner. When arrayed together, these unit cells form a simple orchard with trees in equally spaced rows in two directions.

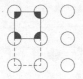

So where is the number five? Perhaps some visual elaboration would have helped here, but Browne announces in his dedicatory epistle that he does not wish to 'affright the common Reader with any other Diagramms'. However, it is possible to superimpose a slightly larger 'unit cell' at forty-five degrees to the first, with one central tree and a quarter share of four new trees at each corner, that does begin to look like a quincunx. But this leads to the same simple orchard when it is repeated.

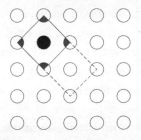

This does not appear to be the arrangement of trees in Cyrus's garden as described by the Greek historian Xenophon, which Browne paraphrases as having 'the rows and orders so handsomely disposed; or five trees so set together, that a regular angularity, and through prospect was left on every side'. This could still be a simple square grid spaced so as to leave good orthogonal and diagonal sightlines, but Browne's description does suggest something more complicated that would give a sense of the trees being laid out in distinct sets of five as well. For a true quincunx to be the repeating unit cell, it turns out that the trees must be set out in rows that cross at every third tree.

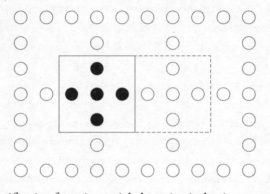

The justification for quincunxial plantation is that it supposedly gives trees more light. In the simple square grid all trees receive the same light, although of course they shade one another if they are too closely planted. If the trees are set out at the same spacing in their rows but with the intersections only at every second tree rather than every tree, the trees at the intersections receive less light than the trees in between. The same goes for the array based on repeating quincunxes, in which the intersections happen at every third tree. Some trees are better off in these arrangements, but some are relatively more shaded. The only answer to planting an orchard to give every tree equal light is to follow the simplest arrangement and to increase the spacing sufficiently. The quincunx is no more than an ornamental conceit.

*

November has come, and it is time for me to plant my own quincunx. I have no plans for a commercial orchard, and so the question of how best to arrange rows of trees for maximum yield does not arise. I buy four bare-root apple trees of interesting varieties and a young pine. I check the dimensions to make sure I have a perfect square and then dig the holes, one in each corner and one in the centre. I tease out the roots of each tree and place it gently in the appropriate hole, filling it with earth and pressing it down as I go. Finally, I stake the trees and lash them together so that they will not be blown over in the next storm. I step back to inspect my naive handiwork. They are not the first trees I have ever planted, but it is the first time I have tried to impose a regular design on nature. I am not sure I like the pattern I have made in a garden that is frankly governed by randomness. I wonder for how long my little plantation will read as a quincunx.

I feel Browne's focus on the quincunx may be a case of 'visual editing' on his part in order to extract maximum interest from the apparently unpromising starting point of the simplest of geometric arrays. It serves him well as he embraces the five-fold in plants and the grid-like patterns on pine cones and catkins. But in essence there is nothing to be explored here except the connections that he imagines. Browne does not give us diagrams or, as he also says, 'mathematicall truths' because he prefers the ambiguous richness of text, the impressed array of words on the page and their infinite possibilities of meaning.

What Browne did not know is that the quincunxial orchard and the five-fold arrangements produced by phyllotaxis do in fact share common cause in a scientific sense. Both are directed towards the same end – that of supplying plants most efficiently with the light and energy they need in order to grow. He might have been disappointed to understand that there is nothing paradisiacal or even biological about this. It is solely the battle between physical forces that governs the emergence of these patterns. He would be consoled, though, to recognize that this in no way removes God from the garden.

I am beginning to think part of my aversion to the garden is based on an unwillingness, inculcated in me by science, to find easy 'wonder' there. If, as Browne claims, the observation of nature in a garden is inimical to atheistic thinking, then perhaps this is the root of my discomfort.

Although he operated on the scientific fringe, Browne's speculations as a **'botanologer'** on symmetry and pattern in plants are pertinent again today, and are now taken further by the new geometry of fractals, in which similar patterns are found to repeat on different scales, for example in the tapering leaves of familiar plants such as ferns as well as in the seed heads studied by Browne.

Phyllotaxis, according to the science writer Philip Ball, 'contains a hidden mathematical pattern for which we are unlikely to find an explanation by rooting around in the genetics of plant developmental biology'. There is something reassuring about this, not so much because it is a poke in the eye for reductionism and the apparently inexorable tendency for discoveries to be made at scales smaller than the visible, as because it restores the idea that simply looking at things in the right way might still have much to teach us. Assisted by computer visualizations, plant biologists are once again finding that observation of the growth and form of plants may be as instructive as analysing their component genes and proteins.

I find a man who I am tempted to characterize as Browne's spiritual successor just outside Norwich at the John Innes Centre. Professor Enrico Coen is a plant geneticist who has made his name in science for a

❁❁❁❁❁❁❁❁❁❁❁❁❁❁❁❁❁❁❁❁❁❁❁

botanologer (GC, 1658) / **botanist** (Miscellany Tracts, 1684): Browne was aware of the need to explain what it was that he and his peers were doing, and this is one of many words he coined to give names to emerging scientific disciplines. *Phytology*, the study of plants, also makes its debut in *The Garden of Cyrus*. In *Religio Medici*, Browne thinks there may be something also in *phytognomy*, the art or science of deducing the qualities of a plant from its appearance (hence the prescribing of asparagus as seventeenth-century Viagra). Other new disciplines or their practitioners include *mineralogist*, *ichthyology*, *zoographer* and *cryptography*, as well as a notable pseudoscience, *rhabdomancy*, meaning divining by means of a rod. Around 1682, in a late note on garlands and the kinds of flowers and plants used in them, Browne improved on *botanologer* by adding the word botanist to the English language.

new understanding of what controls the development of flowers, work for which he was awarded the Darwin Medal of the Royal Society. He also has a fine disregard for the artificial boundaries erected between science and the arts. He is an accomplished portrait painter, often persuading visiting scientists to sit for him. Furthermore, he has just written a visionary book that is sure to provoke more cautious colleagues to critical apoplexy. In *Cells to Civilizations*, Coen aims to identify common factors that organize life at every scale, from the division of biological cells during the growth of organisms to the statelier pace of evolution and the development of human civilization. It is a book of Brownean scope and daring, an attempt to provide the 'theory of everything' that biology seems to lack. Enrico seems to share with Browne the ability to step aside from the trudge of the scientific project and take in a bigger view. He understands that some of his peers may be sceptical or worse, but he is confident that his book will connect nevertheless. 'People who want to see unifying ideas – it will appeal to them,' he says. 'The question is how you do these things in a critical way, and not end up in mystical pondering. I feel I'm doing it in a way that's very grounded in science.'

We meet in one of the gardens slotted in among the John Innes Centre laboratory buildings. It is a hot day and Enrico is wearing a light short-sleeved shirt with a checked pattern that reminds me of Browne's grid of lozenges. The sun glints off his tanned bald head until we take shelter under a rose bower. Everywhere are blossoms. I fear for the stooks of ripe artichoke that stand nearby: 'artichoke omelette' has been written up on a whiteboard as one course of a feast planned for the end of an interdisciplinary seminar of biologists and computer scientists.

Enrico offers welcome evidence to refute the 'two cultures' view of the arts and sciences that has historically bedevilled British education and academia. 'It's all a false dichotomy,' he insists. 'Science tells us important things, but it's also a human activity. We can't separate that.' As if in proof, his oil sketches line the stairwells of the John Innes Centre. One of his portraits is of Jonathan Miller, the physician and theatre director, perhaps the most conspicuous refutation of the two-cultures doctrine at work in Britain. Although Enrico was born in Liverpool, his own breadth of learning must be something to do with his Italian heritage. Both his parents are half-Italian, and both are scientists, but there is an echo of the Renaissance spirit that allows art and science to occupy the same space. 'We used to go to Italy every summer holiday,' he says. 'They would take me to art galleries. I never really grew up with a sharp divide.'

One of Enrico's favourite models for investigating flower shape is the *Antirrhinum* or snapdragon. The snapdragon, as it happens, already has a special connection with the city of Norwich. A snapping dragon was once a feature of medieval religious processions linked to the Guild of St George, although by the time of Thomas Browne it had been incorporated into mayoral ceremonies, where it still makes its appearance today.

It is the asymmetric arrangement of its petals that causes the flower to resemble a dragon's mouth. Exactly how the snapdragon, or any flower, actually develops its distinctive shape is hard to figure. But the regularity of that shape is at the heart of the matter. Pollinating insects – bees in the case of snapdragons – must find the experience of visiting the flower memorable in order to seek out others like it. If its petals vary too much in number, shape or size, the approaching bee may not recognize it or may not be able to gather pollen successfully. Number is especially important, it seems. 'There is an evolutionary tendency for flowers to become more consistent in the numbers of features such as petals,' Enrico tells me.

Before genes were known, naturalists had little option but to classify plants according to the shapes of their leaves and flowers, but they could not say how or why they take the wide variety of forms that they do. Snapdragons are easy to grow and were once a popular model organism in plant breeding experiments, but fell out of fashion when attention turned to crop plants. Later, though, they were found to possess a type of gene that can jump to different positions in the genome and thereby produce mutations. Enrico had a hunch that these genes might be useful tools for investigating flower shape.

In the snapdragon, one gene is responsible for the symmetrical folding back of the petals that happens in most flowers. Another gene breaks that symmetry so that the flower morphs into the familiar dragon's-mouth shape. One of the petals becomes the dragon's 'tongue' and the landing platform for the bee, while the others curl back to make the dragon's 'head'. Without these genetic components, the snapdragon would develop without the petals folding back or with five symmetrical petals like so many other flowers, and it would lose its exclusive appeal

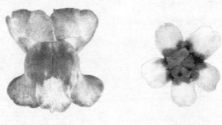

WILD TYPE   PELORIC

to bees. 'The asymmetry of the snapdragon relates to the asymmetry of the bee,' Enrico explains. 'It reflects the fact that it's visited by an animal.' This understanding demanded knowledge of the mechanism of individual genes but also relied on the traditional naturalist's skill of observation. 'It's relating different perspectives. That's how you arrive at understanding.'

Enrico's research today involves a powerful combination of the latest knowledge of plant genetics and the use of computer models to visualize patterns of growth. Members of his team work at large computer screens; there are few growing plants in the lab. But there is beauty. On one of the screens, I see astonishing high-speed sequences of the inner structure of plants taking shape as they grow. They are so perfect and bright that I assume they are computer graphics. But I am corrected: they are assembled from natural images. On other occasions, though, Enrico's team do create entirely artificial visualizations of plant growth. These are based solely on data describing the behaviour of the individual cells that make them up, with no information about overall morphology.

The visualizations are beautiful – Enrico's painter's eye is obvious in some of the illustrations in the team's scientific papers – but also highly instructive. They are a vital aid to help fellow scientists grasp the basic algorithms of growth and a salutary reminder that there's no substitute for seeing. The images are uncannily close to what we see in the garden: they demonstrate in the most graphic way the power of nature to develop complex organisms using a very few, simple rules. Perhaps it is this power that we sense when we observe the splitting of a palm leaf or the lozenges on a catkin.

But actual gardening? 'It's not something I get,' says Enrico.

5
Science

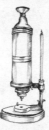

'The wary and evading assertor'

Pseudodoxia Epidemica

IN 1879, AFTER years of research, Leslie Keeley, a former surgeon for the Union Army in the American Civil War, and John Oughton, a pharmacist in the little town of Dwight, Illinois, declared that they had developed a treatment for alcoholism. 'Drunkenness is a disease and I can cure it,' Keeley told the local newspaper. The two men opened a sanatorium in Dwight, where sufferers could check in for the month-long course of treatment, which involved the gradual withdrawal of rations of whiskey and injections four times a day with the 'gold cure'.

Keeley's programme proved popular because it saw alcoholism as a disease rather than a moral weakness. It promised caring treatment in place of ineffectual quack remedies or incarceration in an asylum. The Keeley Institute expanded to more than 200 franchises throughout the United States and in Europe. When the last one closed, as late as 1965, 400,000 people had taken the cure, including '17,000 drunken doctors'.

The medical profession, however, was always sceptical of Keeley's methods, and the composition of his brightly coloured injection liquids – said to be 'bi-chlorides of gold' – remained secret. Today, some historians believe that more gold was administered in the name of medicine by the Keeley institutes than at any time in history; others claim that no gold was ever involved.

From long before the time of Thomas Browne, and sporadically ever since, gold has been thought to possess health-giving properties. Once, alchemists hoped to convert its incorruptible essence into the elixir of life, and even now it is tempting to believe that this unique and precious substance, found rarely but always in its pure state, must have some practical benefit to offer man.

Does gold have any efficacy as a medicine? Did it ever? It is an ideal topic for Browne: it is believed by many that it does, but not by all, and it is hard to establish the truth of the matter by experiment. Browne's discussion of the medicinal merits or otherwise of gold in *Pseudodoxia Epidemica* sets out as the rational enquiry of a physician, but soon expands to allow for a prodigious display of classical and Renaissance learning and fertile philosophical speculation.

Pseudodoxia Epidemica is a long work – some 200,000 words – and it tackles hundreds of vulgar errors. Some Browne discusses at length, others he dispatches in little more than a sentence. His discussion of gold is exemplary. In its six paragraphs, it shows his logical and rhetorical methods to fine effect. Although *Pseudodoxia Epidemica* is written in Browne's plainest English, the rich topic of gold also tempts him to a few enjoyable touches of literary ormolu. All this makes it a rewarding text for close analysis.

I recommend that you read this passage – or any of Browne's writing – out loud. Only then can you feel properly the rhythm of the prose that propels Browne's argument. The sentences are often long, and appear at first to be broken up with many subordinate clauses and much punctuation, but these are aids and not impediments, put there to enhance the metre for the greater pleasure and better comprehension of the reader.

He begins plainly enough with a bald statement of the claim that is popularly made:

That Gold inwardly taken, either in substance, infusion, decoction or extinction, is a cordial of great efficacy, in sundry Medical uses, although a practice much used, is also much questioned, and by no man determined beyond dispute.

Browne takes care to include all the ways he can think of in which gold might be ingested, as a solid (*in substance*), in dissolved form in water or some other liquor (*infusion*), as a concentrate stirred up in hot water (*decoction*), or as the liquor that results when the hot metal is quenched in a liquid (*extinction*). He signals that he will not prejudge the matter at the outset by giving conspicuously equal weight to both practitioners (*much used*) and sceptics (*much questioned*).

Medieval alchemists believed they could exploit the link between the energy-giving sun, its symbolic metal gold, and the human heart (a *cordial* is a liquor thought to be good for the heart, the Latin stem *cor* meaning heart). They made preparations of 'potable gold' by heating gold utensils and then quenching them in wine, although later chemistry has shown that no gold is in fact dissolved by this method. Paracelsus and his followers in the sixteenth century, knowing the secret of aqua regia, the unique mixture of acids that does dissolve gold, promoted remedies that truly did contain the metal (and the charlatans of the day made a killing by pretending the same). Along with other new chemical medicines, gold began to find a place in the pharmacopoeias. Its medicinal utility is thus a matter of some controversy by the time Browne enters the debate.

He proceeds to scope out the range and strength of people's views. By establishing these limits, he opens up a middle ground, where we can already sense that he might settle:

There are hereof I perceive two extream opinions; some excessively magnifying it, and probably beyond its deserts; others extreamly vilifying it, and perhaps below its demerits.

He is assiduous in maintaining the symmetry of the previous sentence that vouches for his impartiality (*excessively magnifying, and probably . . . / extreamly vilifying, and perhaps . . .*). This symmetrical device is deployed once more in the sentence that follows (*Some / others*):

> Some affirming it a powerful Medicine in many diseases, others averring that so used, it is effectual in none:

The repeated use of these balancing phrases does more than advertise Browne's own balance. It also shows the hand of a skilled rhetorician, with his use of the 'rule of three' bringing this opening to a satisfying caesura.

Now we turn a corner:

> and in this number are very eminent Physicians, *Erastus*, *Duretus*, *Rondeletius*, *Brassavolus*, and many other; who beside the strigments and sudorous adhesions from mens hands, acknowledge that nothing proceedeth from Gold in the usual decoction thereof.

For the first time, Browne invokes a number of authorities on one side of the argument only. Often in *Pseudodoxia Epidemica* he will line up appropriate experts whom he respects (from antiquity as well as the Renaissance) on both sides before picking his way through their logic, usually onto some middle ground. Perhaps he is preparing to do the same here. Erastus was a student of Plato; the others are French and Italian physicians of the sixteenth century. Will Browne side with them? He'll need to be persuaded:

> Now the capital reason that led men unto this opinion, was their observation of the inseparable nature of Gold: it being excluded in the same quantity as it was received, without alteration of parts, or diminution of its gravity.

In addition to his appeal to authority, he now offers the additional evidence of experiment. This will allow us to deploy our own sense of reason in weighing the case. Gold is indeed profoundly unreactive, as Browne says. Observed not to undergo change in the world (*inseparable*), why should it then be believed that it undergoes change in the human body? And if *it* does not change, then surely it cannot exert a change on the body in return. Browne's scientific mind here anticipates certain basic principles of physics and chemistry which will not be clearly set out for another century or so, such as the law of conservation of mass and the rule that one chemical element cannot be changed into another.

With his next paragraph, Browne prepares us for the fact that he will not be aligning himself precisely with the scholars he has cited, even though he agrees with them as far as their observation goes that gold is not altered by the human digestive system:

> Now herein to deliver somewhat which in a middle way may be entertained; we first affirm, that the substance of Gold is invincible by the powerfullest action of natural heat; and that not only alimentally in a substantial mutation, but also medicamentally in any corporeal conversion.

It is notable, in the light of Browne's careful symmetry earlier on, that he does not stop to name these opposing voices who are now pulling him away from Erastus and the rest towards his *middle way*. Paracelsus's ideas of chemical medicine were still considered radical at this time, and it may be that Browne does not wish to 'out' himself to his fellow physicians as a Paracelsian.* Instead, we will shortly be asked to think of

---

* Kevin Faulkner draws my attention to Browne's coffin-plate, the last few words of which read: 'Corporis spagyricci pulvere plumbum in aurum convertit'. Spagyric is a Paracelsian term referring to the manufacture of medicine by (al)chemical methods. Translation might run: 'By the dust of his spagyric body he converts lead into gold,' although the auriferous aspect of alchemy would have been the least of Browne's reasons for interest in it.

gold in a more subtle way, distinguishing between its *substance* and other, more tenuous qualities. First, though, Browne piles on more evidence that gold is not altered by passage through the body:

> As is very evident, not only in the swallowing of golden bullets, but in the lesser and foliate divisions thereof: passing the stomach and guts even as it doth the throat, that is, without abatement of weight or consistence. So that it entereth not the veins with those electuaries, wherein it is mixed: but taketh leave of the permeant parts, at the mouths of the *Meseraicks*, or Lacteal Vessels, and accompanieth the inconvertible portion unto the siege. Nor is its substantial conversion expectible in any composition or aliment wherein it is taken.

Browne cannot resist deploying his physician's jargon in this bravura display of his own expert knowledge (an *electuary* is a medicinal paste; the *Meseraicks* are the intestines). After blinding his readers with science, he quickly lifts their spirits with a joke and an entertaining reminder of the consequences of his reasoning for some familiar stories of golden transformations:

> And therefore that was truly a starving absurdity, which befel the wishes of *Midas*. And little credit there is to be given to the golden Hen, related by *Wendlerus*.

He now concludes his opening argument with a clear restatement of the part of the problem that he has chosen to isolate – that gold is essentially immutable – and the barest hint that there might nevertheless be other ways that it can exert an effect on the body without chemical transformation. This is something that his readers who are up to date with the latest science may already have begun to guess:

So in the extinction of Gold, we must not conceive it
parteth with any of its salt or dissoluble principle thereby, as we may
affirm of Iron; for the parts thereof are fixed beyond division, nor
will they separate upon the strongest test of fire.

The comparison with iron is carefully chosen. It is not only that
this metal provides a chemical contrast with gold: iron readily forms
compounds likely to have an effect on the body, for example. He has
chosen iron (and not, say, copper) for a specific reason that his scientifically educated readers may once again be able to guess.

This second paragraph ends with a coda that further serves to put us
on our guard:

This we affirm of
pure Gold: for that which is currant and passeth in stamps amongst
us, by reason of its allay, which is a proportion of Silver or Copper
mixed therewith, is actually dequantitated by fire, and possibly by
frequent extinction.

In other words, all that glisters is not gold, and Browne's arguments
apply to pure gold only, not to baser materials that might be called gold
in casual discourse, or hawked as gold by charlatans, or naively thought
to be gold by ordinary people.

With his third paragraph, Browne now reveals the dramatic twist to
which he has been leading:

Secondly, Although the substance of Gold be not immuted or
its gravity sensibly decreased, yet that from thence some vertue may
proceed either in substantial reception or infusion we cannot safely
deny.

This is new. Now he tells us that he believes – or at least does not
wholly disbelieve – that gold might exert an effect after all, even if it

is itself unchanged. It seems like a direct contradiction of what he has already told us. But he has evidence that such may be the case in principle: the 'vulgar errors' that precede this one in *Pseudodoxia Epidemica*, 'the Loadstone' and 'Bodies Electrical', concern the new phenomena of magnetism and **electricity**. The section on the lodestone is the longest

✤✤✤✤✤✤✤✤✤✤ ✤ ✤ ✤✤✤✤✤✤✤✤✤✤✤

electricity (PE, 1646): Browne's lithe visual imagination yields him some uncanny insights into these mysterious new phenomena. Drawing an analogy with the circular motion observed when one blows on motes of dust in sunlight, he gives us a compelling picture of electric field lines that would not be properly mapped until Michael Faraday's work two centuries later. He all but gives a statement of the inverse square law of magnetic and electrical attractions: 'a tenuous emanation or continued effluvium, which after some distance retracteth into it self'. Ice, he intuits correctly, is generally less transparent than crystals of salt or saltpetre because 'Its atoms are not concreted into continuity'.

For many of his readers, this is their first chance to understand the new discoveries about magnetism set out (in Latin) by William Gilbert's *De Magnete* of 1600. (Indeed, a large part of Browne's project in *Pseudodoxia Epidemica* is to present in ordinary English knowledge both ancient and modern previously only available in Latin.) But they have the added spice of Browne's own confirmatory experiments. One of these Browne devised in order to challenge the belief that two needles stroked with the same magnet would point to the same letter of the alphabet when set to pivot at the centre of respective abecedary circles. 'The conceit is excellent, and if the effect would follow, somewhat divine,' Browne marvels. He can see how a pair of such devices might work like a wireless telegraph. But will they? He constructs two circles of wood, which he marks with the letters of the alphabet. He then takes two needles made of the same steel and touched with the same magnet. He places the two wheels close to one another and moves the needle of one of them. The other does not respond; it stands unmoved 'like *Hercules* pillars'. He cannot disguise his disappointment. But ocular proof and reason prevail, and he reasons further that the devices would not work for sending messages in any case as the movement of the needle from A to B on one wheel would be echoed by an *opposing* rotation, that is from A to Z, on the other.

Explaining invisible phenomena is one of the urgent tasks for early modern scientists. In 1646, it is magnetism, electricity, and the worlds at different scales made visible for the first time by the invention of the telescope and the microscope. Soon, it will be Newton on gravity and light.

Browne makes the first use in English of the word 'electricity' when he writes that 'Crystal will calefie unto electricity', in other words that a suitable material when rubbed and warmed by friction will acquire a static electrical charge. He goes on to puzzle as to why only some materials behave in this way, and what the respective properties are that the attractor and the attracted bodies must possess, and what it is that actually passes between them when this happens.

of all, a veritable essay on the mysteries of magnetism. If iron can exert strange forces, cannot gold too?

For possible it is that bodies may emit vertue and operation without abatement of weight; as is evident in the Loadstone, whose effluencies are continual, and communicable without a minoration of gravity.

If crystals and amber can do this, can gold too?

And the like is observable in Bodies electrical, whose emissions are less subtile. So will a Diamond or Saphire emit an effluvium sufficient to move the Needle or a Straw, without diminution of weight. Nor will polished Amber although it send forth a gross and corporal exhalement, be found a long time defective upon the exactest scales. Which is more easily conceivable in a continued and tenacious effluvium, whereof a great part retreats into its body.

With these two examples of weird physical phenomena where the substance exerting the effect does not appear to change, Browne throws open the doors of possibility. How wide dare he push them? Do even the amulets that the superstitious wear to ward off evil have some real action?

Thirdly, If amulets do work by emanations from their bodies, upon those parts whereunto they are appended, and are not yet observed to abate their weight; if they produce visible and real effects by imponderous and invisible emissions, it maybe unjust to deny the possible efficacy of Gold, in the non-omission of weight, or deperdition of any ponderous particles.

Steady, Tom. Elsewhere, Browne has given short shrift to amulets when they are falsely sold as cures for diseases and have no effect at all. Now, he uses this vulgar error as grist to his own mill: if you believe in amulets, he says, you must at least stop to consider the possibility that gold might act by means of similar *imponderous and invisible emissions*.

Browne's open-mindedness is not only commendable, it also seems remarkably foresighted. We are now accustomed to the use of radioactive isotopes in cancer therapy – 'powerful Medicine' acting without 'diminution of its gravity'. Indeed, metallic gold-198 has been used against some tumours because its short radioactive half-life of 2.7 days in combination with its chemical inertness means it is safe to leave in the patient's body.

Browne's final analogy bears up less well to twenty-first-century scrutiny, however:

> Lastly, Since *Stibium* or Glass of Antimony, since also its *Regulus* will manifestly communicate unto Water or Wine, a purging and vomitory operation; and yet the body it self, though after iterated infusions, cannot be found to abate either vertue or weight: we shall not deny but Gold may do the like, that is, impart some effluences unto the infusion, which carry with them the separable subtilties thereof.

It is known now that a tiny quantity of antimony does dissolve in such infusions even though the regulus, the crystal of the pure element, from which it comes appears unchanged. Antimony was widely used in medicine in medieval and early modern medicine; physicians even prescribed pills made of it as reusable laxatives because so little was lost on each use. Browne now moves to his summing up:

> That therefore this Metal thus received, hath any undeniable effect, we shall not imperiously determine, although beside the former experiments, many more may induce us to believe it.

Clearing the brushwood of caveats and double negatives in this sentence, we discover that Browne basically wishes to reserve judgement: he's not prepared to say that gold *isn't* effective as medicine; but neither, on the strength of these analogies and experiments, can he assert with complete confidence that it is. It is a typical (or perhaps I should say not untypical) Brownean conclusion, open-minded to a fault, but also intriguingly open-ended. Now, he has more practical advice to impart:

> But since the point is dubious and not yet authentically decided, it will be no discretion to depend on disputable remedies; but rather in cases of known danger, to have recourse unto medicines of known and approved activity.

It is the standard advice of doctors down the ages: stick to the tried and trusted medicine. But Browne also has a more far-reaching point to make:

> For, beside the benefit accruing unto the sick, hereby may be avoided a gross and frequent errour, commonly committed in the use of doubtful remedies, conjointly with those which are of approved vertues; that is to impute the cure unto the conceited remedy, or place it on that whereon they place their opinion. Whose operation although it be nothing, or its concurrence not considerable, yet doth it obtain the name of the whole cure: and carrieth often the honour of the capital energie, which had no finger in it.

That is to say, there is a danger that, if enough people start taking gold, then gold comes to be seen as a 'cure' even if it actually has no effect: so many people can't be wrong. Except, of course, they can. And their persistence in being wrong then blocks the introduction of genuine remedies. This *gross and frequent errour* is still with us, seen for example in the indiscriminate prescribing of antibiotics in response to public demand.

Browne ends with a sentence that seems very familiar to us now – the scientist's habitual refrain that 'more research is needed'. But he is once again in the vanguard of what seventeenth-century medical practice might be. This is nothing less than a call for clinical trials of potable gold:

> Herein exact and critical trial should be made by publick enjoinment, whereby determination might be setled beyond debate: for since thereby, not only the bodies of men, but great Treasures might be preserved, it is not only an errour of Physick, but folly of State, to doubt thereof any longer.

What kind of reader does Browne have in mind here? Make no mistake: he is serious about his mission. To Browne – and especially to Browne the medical materialist, mindful that there are always people on the streets of Norwich hawking false remedies – errors are worse even than heresies because they can do real harm to other people. Yet he is moderate in his argument. He is open to all possibilities and even-handed in his consideration of them. He makes it clear that he is drawing upon his learning, both general and as a medical specialist, but is not academic. He gives his reasoning and cites his sources. He takes the occasion to enlighten his readers in regard to some new science and even throws in some amusing sidelights that may cause them to think more critically about some popular fables.

Here, as in most of the vulgar errors that he addresses in *Pseudodoxia Epidemica*, Browne appeals to authority, ancient and modern, to the powers of reason and reasonableness, and to the power of **deductive**

❖❖❖❖❖❖❖❖❖❖ ❖ ❖❖ ❖❖❖❖❖❖❖❖❖❖

deductive (PE, 1646): Although he coins the word as a loose synonym for 'derivative' or 'lesser', its more precise meaning in logic is established in time for the later editions of *Pseudodoxia Epidemica*. Deductive reasoning proceeds logically from statements of the known truth towards conclusions that must therefore also be true. By contrast, inductive reasoning reaches general conclusions from specific cases, but these can never be certain and are always subject to falsification. Deduction is robust in method, logic. Such a combination could be very dry, but Browne takes care to ensure that it is not so. A favourite example of mine is his examination of the legend reported by Herodotus that Xerxes's army during its eastward march into Greece in 480 BCE 'drank whole rivers dry'. A plodding mind might have demanded to know the size of this army, the volume of these rivers, and so on, before calculating an answer. But Browne cuts straight through the problem with unassailable logic, finding it 'wondrous strange, that they exhausted not the provision of the Countrey, rather then the waters thereof'.

Browne is always aware of the requirements for scientific proof – that extraordinary claims require extraordinary evidence, that a single contrary demonstration is sufficient to demolish a hypothesis – but this burden is lightly borne, often expounded with a story rather than a lecture. Disproving the unlikely belief that lions are scared of cockerels, for example, Browne simply cites a story he has heard recently that when a lion belonging to the Prince of Bavaria escaped into a neighbour's yard it ate his cockerels and hens too, notwithstanding their bravery.

Though he does not on this occasion imbibe a cordial of gold, Browne performs his own experiments, as we have seen already with the unbooming bittern and the kingfisher weathervane. Do earwigs have wings? He prises aside the wing case to prove they do. Do flies buzz by some means other than using their mouths? He decapitates flies and

---

but can yield disappointingly feeble results. Induction is inherently fragile, but capable of leaping to great revelations. Deduction is satisfying to the mind, induction is unsettling.

Aristotle was the father of deductive logic. Francis Bacon founded the inductive method, though he was always dissatisfied with its manifest imperfection. Browne defers explicitly to Aristotle in his writing, but owes more to the experimentalism of Bacon, as his investigations with his bittern attest. Although Browne's bittern never boomed, he knows that absence of evidence is not evidence of absence, and so he holds off reporting his experience until a friend – one of a number whom he seems to have commissioned to go about the reed beds of the county – can say that he has seen the bird booming while standing clear of surrounding vegetation. From this trustworthy observation, he was finally able to draw the certain conclusion that bitterns boom without help from the reeds. Deduction wins over induction.

finds that they buzz still. '[D]iscursive enquiry and rationall conjecture' are all very well, he writes at the end of *The Garden of Cyrus*. But 'sense and ocular Observation' are what's needed to strike the 'dispatching blows unto errour'. Although it is Francis Bacon who is usually credited with the invention of the experimental method in science, it is likely that Browne did more actual experiments, and he even dares to refute Bacon when he repeats an investigation in which iron is dissolved in aqua fortis (nitric acid). Bacon finds that the overall weight of the reactants remains constant, even though copious noxious fumes are given off, but Browne correctly records a loss in weight. Browne's experiments were in turn occasionally repeated by notable successors, such as Robert Boyle, the first modern chemist, who took three attempts to confirm Browne's claim that aqua fortis can cause oil to coagulate. Browne's standing as an experimental scientist should need no greater confirmation than this.

Sometimes, an experiment fails, and Browne endears himself to the reader by saying so. His candid reporting brings a fresh kind of authority to his resolution of vulgar errors. These are experiments any reader can imagine doing for himself – or can now that Browne has put the idea in his head, for it almost certainly will not have occurred to him before. The very idea of an experiment designed in order to establish a scientific fact is quite new. Yet Browne is offering a life lesson here. Some of his harshest criticism in *Pseudodoxia Epidemica* is reserved for those who persist in believing dubious things even though they possess the power of reason and the wherewithal to do the experiment that would establish the truth of the matter; these people, says Browne, fail 'in the intention of man it self'. Man, in other words, has a God-given duty to experiment.

Unpublished notes provide raw details of many more experiments that Browne conducted lifelong. They range widely and wildly in their topics, showing evidence of the curious mind more than any ordered proto-scientific drive to pursue an investigation to its conclusion. All is urgency, but which way to go? Browne is conscious of the opportunity, after centuries of ignorance, 'to erect a new *Britannia*', and that it is scientific knowledge that will help to do this, though as a believer in the End of Days he is aware too that 'time may be too short for our designes'. This sense of a race against time – a race with the hurdles of people's wilful ignorance in the way – is widely shared among the curious elite. John Evelyn, for example, hails Browne as one of the 'society of learned and ingenuous men…by whome we might hope to redeeme the tyme that has bin lost, in pursuing vulgar errours'.

Some of these hatchling ideas Browne nurtures for later inclusion in essays for publication. Others find their way into correspondence with the more professional set of natural philosophers of the Royal Society in London or with like-minded gentleman-scholars on their Norfolk estates. The traffic is two-way: Browne keeps abreast of the latest scientific developments, learning promptly, for example, of Leeuwenhoek's discovery of spermatozoa, 'finding such a vast number of little animals in the melt of a cod, or the liquor which runnes from it…that they much exceed the number of men upon the whole earth at one time'.

Most, though, are extempore notes for his own education. One important recurrent theme is the generation of plants and animals. Browne notes with wonder the ability of plants to regenerate from their roots or even ashes. But his most significant contribution to scientific knowledge may come from his experiments on eggs. Living in Norfolk rather than in London, he was arguably better situated than fellows of the Royal Society to procure a variety of live eggs for experimental purposes. Browne studied the effect of heat and the action of substances such as vinegar and saltpetre on the eggs of chickens, frogs and skates. Joseph Needham's view was that these first explorations of the chemical constitution of eggs

show Sir Thomas to have been more than simply the supreme artist in English prose, which is his common title to remembrance… The only conclusion that can be drawn from these remarkable observations is that it was in the 'elaboratory' in Sir Thomas' house at Norwich that the first experiments in chemical embryology were undertaken. His significance in this connection has been quite overlooked, and it is time to recognise that his originality and genius in this field shows itself to be hardly less remarkable than in so many others.

In these enquiries into the nature of materials and what passes between them, Browne takes us back to a period in science when unknowns were all around and yet could be probed with relative ease. We too easily forget this today, and allow ourselves to think these enquiries silly. Yet how would we set about one of these investigations even now if suddenly obliged to unlearn so much of what we have learnt since the seventeenth century?

How are vulgar errors handled in the twenty-first century? Ben Goldacre's book *Bad Science* is arguably the most constructive among a rash of books that have recently sought to shine the light of reason and science on some of the popular misunderstandings to which we are still alarmingly prone. He does not detain his readers on the medicinal merits of gold cordial, although he does take thirty-five pages to deal with the scientifically simpler, but presently hotly contested, question of homoeopathy.

He declares at the outset that he is 'not desperately interested' in alternative medicine. Instead, he wishes to use homoeopathy as a kind of case study to examine how it is in science and medicine that we know if an action produces the results claimed for it. This has relevance beyond the eccentric backwater of homoeopathy because mainstream drug-based medicine – 'big pharma' – surrounds itself with a similar mythology of miraculous pills that may be nothing like as effective as even doctors are led to believe. Goldacre wishes to give us the critical faculties to appraise claims made for health-giving properties whatever their provenance.

I won't deconstruct the whole of Goldacre's argument as I have done for Browne's gold. He continues with a brief history of homoeopathy, together with a statement of its principles – that 'like cures like', and that very great dilutions of the supposedly active ingredient are more effective than a concentrated dose. Goldacre debunks the dilution principle using simple arithmetic to expose its absurdity. Then he comes to the nub: homoeopathic patients say the treatment makes them feel better. The truth of this claim is almost impossible to assess (as it is for some conventional medicines) because of the placebo effect and because patients may simply get better anyway. In the end, Goldacre surprises us and concedes, Browne-like, that 'going to see a homeopath is probably a helpful intervention, in some cases, for some people, even if the pills are just placebos', although he remains far less forgiving of the pseudoscientific foldcrol with which the homoeopathy industry defends its interests.

The major difference in the way that Goldacre tackles this example of twenty-first-century pseudoscience lies in his tone. Beneath his rigorous dismantling of the 'science' of homoeopathy, there is a sharpness that edges into superciliousness. Although he tries hard to maintain a dispassionate balance, he cannot altogether disguise his impatience with the whole enterprise, and occasionally a mocking undercurrent cannot help but break the surface. 'This is another universe of foolishness,' he explodes at one point.

Goldacre is a model of restraint compared to some other champions of reason. Simon Singh was taken to court for libel by the British Chiropractic Association when he wrote in an article in the *Guardian* in 2008 (promoting his newly published book *Trick or Treatment? Alternative Medicine on Trial*) that the organization 'happily promotes bogus treatments'. In the hearing, the judge ruled that the word 'bogus' had been used as a statement of fact rather than being fair comment, and that it could be taken as meaning 'deliberately false', and was therefore defamatory to the BCA.

Others judge that open ridicule is the best weapon. Francis Wheen includes homoeopathy in a very British attack on dodgy ideas ranging from structuralism to religious fundamentalism. His title says it all: *How Mumbo-Jumbo Conquered the World*. But impatience with the world's foolishness quickly becomes intolerance. Sense about Science, a lobby group which campaigns for better presentation of scientific evidence, has a subsidiary group called Voice of Young Science, whose bright idea it was a few years ago to style themselves 'warriors against claptrap'. Richard Dawkins rails that the irrational views of 'dim losers' now find a ready outlet on the Internet. Mark Henderson's bestselling polemic *The Geek Manifesto*, which argues for a greater role for science in policy-making, is predicated on a tribal world of 'geeks' who find it 'cool to think' and everybody else who apparently doesn't. The Twitter biography of Adam Rutherford, a science writer and broadcaster and one of the editors of the journal *Nature*, is: 'Back off. I'm a scientist.' Even allowing for a degree of ironic self-awareness, it's hardly an invitation to dialogue.

My difficulty is not with the substance of the topics that these and other scientists choose to debate. I am a supporter of evolutionary theory, I think horoscopes are nonsense, I think manufacturers who make **fallaciously** scientific claims for their products should be restrained from doing so, and I am sceptical in various degrees towards homoeopathy, chiropractic, reflexology and acupuncture.

My problem is with the tone – arrogant yet embattled, pious yet aggrieved, seeking to sound authoritative yet coming out so shrill. Why, I ask Mark Henderson, has science come to speak like this? The author of *The Geek Manifesto* is also head of communications at the Wellcome Trust, which annually disburses more than £1 billion in medical and

---

fallaciously (PE, 2nd ed., 1650): In the preface to *Pseudodoxia Epidemica*, Browne writes: 'we are not Magisterial in opinions, nor have we Dictator-like obtruded our conceptions; but in the humility of Enquiries or disquisitions, have only proposed them unto more ocular discerners.' In other words, he stands ready to be refuted by superior observation. Such is his confidence in his own powers that Browne is even prepared to take on any pen 'that shall fallaciously refute us'. This may be a pre-emptive strike against men such as Alexander Ross, the one-time chaplain-in-ordinary to Charles I, who criticized Browne's *Religio Medici* in *Medicus Medicatus*. The feud would continue in 1652, when Ross responded to the publication of *Pseudodoxia Epidemica* with a series of absurd counterclaims such as one denying that a magnet attracts iron.

bioscience research funding. Sitting in the atrium of its sleek modern headquarters, it is absurd to believe that science is on the back foot. Mark nevertheless defends the present rhetoric. 'The more strident end of the standing-up-for-science spectrum, while not always helpful, has its uses,' he tells me. 'They've had an important influence in changing the centre of gravity. They've made it easier for more moderate voices themselves to be seen as not extreme.' Maybe. I have a feeling that a more civil tone might have got us all here sooner.

The difference between pseudoscientific claims made in Thomas Browne's time and those made today does not primarily lie with the improbability of the phenomenon described, or in the plausibility of the claimants, but in the certitude with which the basic science is known. Scientists can now show, for example, that a homoeopathic remedy diluted in the approved manner – thirty times by a factor of a hundred each time – will contain not even one molecule of the supposed active compound. This confidence leads some into arrogance, whereas when less was known – or less was thought known – there was both greater ignorance and greater humility. Browne dare not aver that gold has no effect on the human body, even though the metal passes unchanged through it, because he has learnt of recent discoveries where strange effects are observed without substantial change to the thing exerting the effect. In the circumstances, he reserves making final judgement.

In a climate of more certain science, it seems it is less easy to forgive those who cannot be bothered to understand some of the basics or who purposely ignore the facts and prefer to believe something else entirely. And because foolish beliefs these days are spread not only by harmless gossips, but also by powerful vested interests and by a press whose journalists should (and often in fact do) know better, this merely adds to the frustration. This might still matter little if it were only an ignorable minority of eccentrics who held erroneous thoughts and a minority of quacks who preyed on them. But it is not this way. The fact that the UK National Health Service funds some homoeopathy centres, for example, takes public money away from treating patients with conventional medicines. This gives us all a stake in the matter whether we want it or not.

The word that early modern historians favour to describe the growing discourse between like-minded intellectuals at this time is 'civility'. Hobbesian civility sought a utopian remodelling towards a society in which deference and politeness and sound government would be guarantees against violence and disorder. Baconian civility extended these ideals to the community of natural philosophers as the best means of assuring the furtherance of knowledge and its dissemination in the wider world.

During the English Civil War, when *Pseudodoxia Epidemica* was first published, and afterwards, during the years of the Commonwealth and into the Restoration, when it appeared in five subsequent editions, the notion of civility in general society was tested almost to destruction. For Browne, intellectual chaos and the social chaos were tellingly linked. The times made manifest the confusion and decline that can follow from believing the wrong things. He finds solace in the order displayed in the germination of 'the first two seminall leaves' of plants, but is disturbed that it is so soon lost in the chaotic tangle of their later growth. Even the possibility of knowing has been compromised. England is now the garden after the Fall where 'a Paradise, or unthorny place of knowledge' can no longer be hoped for or achieved.

Yet Browne is interested in thorns, too. His roving mind at first seems rather different from scientists' minds now. Scientists are specialists, and to be a specialist you must focus very narrowly within your chosen field. The greatest scientists, however, are still those with hungry eyes and an omnivorous appetite, curious about everything, keen to find connections. Browne's experiments and observations encompass botany, zoology, biology, chemistry, physics, astronomy, archaeology and anthropology. But, because these disciplines of science are not yet defined, he is also at liberty to range well beyond any of them into areas that many scientists now would consider unworthy of serious attention. 'I am, I confesse, naturally inclined to that, which misguided zeale termes superstition', he writes in *Religio Medici*. What does he mean? Who are these misguided zealots? There must already be persons more outspoken than he against superstitious beliefs, men who are in fact rather more like many of today's scientists. Unlike them, Browne is willing – indeed eager – to take the time to consider the nature of superstition and to try to understand those who are superstitious rather than dismissing them as fools.

He cannot resist 'irregularities, contradictions, and antinomies'. Often, he will let a silly belief go as long as it is one that does not have the full force of an error and does no injury to God. The fact that people believe it amuses him certainly, encourages him in his own sense of superiority perhaps, but more importantly also serves to maintain him in alertness to the real nature of people, which is something that scientists then and now are sometimes apt to forget.

This forbearance is a weakness in the eyes of more rigorous investigators. Browne can never join the emerging community of scientists. He is too much of a prelapsarian: his true wish is not to expand learning but 'to reduce it as it lay at first in a few and solid Authours, and to condemne to the fire those swarms and millions of Rhapsodies, begotten onely to distract and abuse the weaker judgements of Scholars, and to maintaine the Trade and Mystery of Typographers'.

Are not most of us now scientific rationalists, and inclined in our turn to see Browne as one of those superfluous rhapsodists whose words are at risk of the flames? Yet our newspapers still print horoscopes, our shops sell 'healing' crystals, our homoeopaths and chiropractors and reflexologists thrive on the custom they receive from willing clients. Even water divining – 'Rhabdomancy' as Browne terms it, 'a fruitless exploration, strongly scenting of *Pagan* derivation' – has been used in the twenty-first century by at least one of Britain's privatized water companies.

Early on, Browne sees that truth is fundamentally slippery. Comparing historical accounts by different authors, he finds that a true version of events is not to be had. Comparing events he has witnessed with his own eyes against later accounts of the same, he finds them at variance.

Nothing can be trusted. The past is no more reliable than the future. There is no simple truth.

Even in science. In his medical practice, he makes do very well with the Galenic concept of the four humours, already 1,500 years old, yet soon after his death to be utterly superseded by new breakthroughs in chemistry and biology. He is aware of the theory of Copernicus, already a century old but slow to spread, that the earth orbits around the sun. The books in his library are all but unanimous, however, that the sun goes round the earth. (He only later acquired Galileo's *Dialogue Concerning the Two Chief World Systems*.) Browne is no Copernican, but nor is he an 'anti-Copernican' – he simply has no informed basis for a conclusive view one way or the other.

He certainly has no fundamental religious objection to heliocentrism. He is always more than happy to decentre man in his universe, though he tends to do it not by juggling the solar system, but by drawing on his great knowledge of the natural world. To the vulgar error that man uniquely stands erect the better to behold the heavens, for example, he reminds us of the *Uranoscopus* genus of fishes, the stargazers, which don't even have to crick their necks to do this. Though never able to read his own, he credits that palms may be read – and sees no reason why, if so, palm-reading should not be valid for any creature with naked forepaws, such as moles and monkeys.

I am making a postmodern point, maybe, one that many scientists might resist even now. Yet it is worth remembering that great scientists, even whole orthodoxies of science, can turn out to have been wrong.

What are scientists wrong about today? And who can we expect to tell us? For scientists today do not often remind us of their own errors, and are loath to expose the fact that backtracking on a once cherished, now disproved theory can be just as humanly painful for them as it is for those in politics or business.

The civility of Browne's day that allowed natural philosophers to engage in dialogue with other scholars of all kinds has been superseded by a grammar largely private to science. A scientific communication must establish its priority, persuade others, and undo rivals. It might also have to please funding agencies, demonstrate 'relevance', and offer itself up for explication to the public. These rhetorical requirements mean that the open, generous and uncomplicated manner of communicating that is natural to many scientists is being forced out by a language that is carefully calibrated, even 'spun'. As science has expanded, the community of natural philosophers and gentleman-scientists building knowledge through civil exchange has been superseded by a profession of specialists who spend most of their time communicating with others like themselves, for whom explaining to the world what they do is often seen as a burdensome duty.

This withdrawal from society produces some odd effects. It induces a state of mind in which isolation becomes an ideal rather than an unfortunate by-product, and in which the only conversation that is acceptable is the one that takes place on the scientific plane. It never would have occurred to Browne, as it does to some more sociopathic scientists today, to suggest that only those with scientific training should have the right to comment on science policy, for example. He would have been distressed, I think, to discover there are scientists today who feel no obligation to understand the non-scientific mind, and who will therefore never comprehend – far less forgive – those credulous souls who pursue irrational customs. They will never turn their minds towards these people for long enough even to consider them as a problem in science, let alone to learn that they behave in the way they do often for quite rational reasons (to gain sympathy, to enjoy social contact, to experience touch, to compensate for being failed by conventional treatment).

How did we arrive in this unhappy place? The Second World War made plain humankind's debt to technology and to the science that underpins it. Electronic devices, plastics, antibiotics and much else were the dividend of that war. At the same time, the dropping of the atomic bomb sent a message that scientific advance was not an unalloyed good. The ride since then has been a bumpy one. Many academics have retraced the path in leisurely detail; I can only point out some of the main sights and the potholes along the way.

In Britain, C. P. Snow's infamous 1959 essay on 'the two cultures' sounded the call to arms. Snow was accurate in diagnosing a problem – that the governing classes, largely educated in the humanities, were ill equipped to rule on matters of science. Merely articulating this fact seemed to exacerbate the problem, however, and battle lines soon hardened between science and the humanities. A series of crises – the thalidomide scandal, the poorly judged attempt to introduce genetically modified crops, the MMR–autism scare, waves of food-borne infections – intensified public hostility towards scientific hauteur.

In 1985, a belated initiative of UK national science associations called for greater 'public understanding of science'. A number of leading universities appointed professors of the public understanding of science, whose pious pronouncements often only antagonized their intended audience. In one memorable outburst, two of these appointees, Richard Dawkins and John Durant, aimed their fire at *The X-Files* television series, which they felt was a public danger for glamorizing pseudoscience.

This first generation of professors has now been succeeded by a more amiable (and telegenic) crew, and the strategic emphasis has been subtly shifted away from 'public understanding of science' to 'public engagement with science' (implying that scientists might actually deign to listen as well as pontificate). Lately, too, an unpredicted and improbable alliance has grown up between scientists in the media and celebrity comedians, which has probably done more to improve the image of science than any official initiative ever could.

In the United States, the postwar journey has followed a somewhat similar path, though with its own milestones (*Sputnik*, DDT, Alar, the Three Mile Island nuclear accident, the *Challenger* disaster). Faith in technological progress remains high and the public perception of science has never reached the lows it reached in Britain – thanks in part to charismatic spokesmen such as Richard Feynman and Carl Sagan, who were able to communicate both the wonder of science and the fact that scientists have broader social responsibilities. Nevertheless, American science has had to contend with its own difficulties, chief among them the fundamentalist Christian opposition to Darwinian evolution.

These trials are hardly enough to justify the portrayal of science as threatened or embattled. Science is in fact winning all down the line. Research funding is often protected when other government spending is cut. 'Popular science' is a thriving genre in book publishing. Science festivals are proliferating. More television programmes have more science content than ever before – not only those designated as science documentaries, but including many devoted to natural history, archaeology, health and other matters.

Those broadly supportive of science – whether qualified scientists or camp followers – have found a collective voice. Now, when something broadly perceived as pseudoscience is given a platform by an organization ostensibly dedicated to scientific ideas, it is liable to be taken to task for the transgression. The Technology, Entertainment and Design conference franchise discovered this when it scheduled a lecture by the parapsychology theorist Rupert Sheldrake; so did the Royal College of Physicians when it allowed a homoeopaths' organization to book its conference facilities. An online survey asking for comments on whether an NHS hospital should refer patients for homoeopathic treatment, which once would have been expected to garner mainly supportive responses from healthcare professionals and homoeopaths, is now quickly shared among sceptics and rationalists who respond with a very different message. Sense about Science has been able to move from naming celebrities who believe silly things (Madonna's valiant efforts to 'neutralize radiation'; Gwyneth Paltrow's dedication to 'biological foods') to praising them when they say something sensible.

These are small victories, but there are greater gains too. I mentioned that Simon Singh was sued for libel by the British Chiropractic Association, but did not add that this case was later overturned on appeal, and became instrumental in securing long overdue reforms of British libel law. Other cases have similarly redounded on the anti-scientific interests that brought them. In short, it is hard to believe that pseudoscience has ever been debunked as thoroughly, enthusiastically and forcefully as it is today.

And yet, are today's po-faced champions of science missing something? Their hope for a day when we all bask in the light of scientific understanding (and never watch *The X-Files*) is surely unrealistic. For, like the poor, the credulous are always with us. But do the credulous in fact know something the rest of us don't? Is a world where some people believe that the stars govern their lives and that there are fairies at the bottom of the garden somehow richer than one where nobody does, where nobody in fact believes anything unless it has a demonstrable base of evidence? Even science cannot advance without that first suspension of rationality needed to admit the imaginative possibility that something unproven might yet be so. They may be foolishly misguided in their specific belief (that diluting something to water intensifies its curative powers, that manipulating one part of the body can heal another), but perhaps they do serve an essential social purpose. Credulousness is surely a natural human behaviour, an expression of empathy at the moment when a myth is passed from one person to another: *I wish to understand you, and I am prepared to demonstrate this by first believing you.* This cannot be a sham. To pretend to believe would not be an empathetic response. The credulous further remind us that beyond the known lies the yet unknown. Albeit unwittingly, they provide a salutary reminder – one that does not issue often enough from scientists' mouths – that science does not have all the answers, that it might even in fact have rather few of them. 'Very beautiful is the Rain-bow' still, writes Browne, after some sentences in *Pseudodoxia Epidemica* summarizing the optical conditions that produce it.

More than a few of Browne's seventeenth-century pseudodoxies are still unresolved. One puzzle, then already familiar, had been examined by Aristotle, Bacon and Descartes: the belief that hot water freezes faster than cold. Browne is happy to overturn these authorities, and agrees with a more recent experimenter that it does not. Since 1969, it has been known as the Mpemba effect, after Erasto Mpemba, a Tanzanian student who stumped a visiting physics lecturer with the problem when he visited his school. From time to time, somebody is moved to investigate the matter and a paper appears in a scientific journal. Half a dozen explanations have recently been proffered, but none has yet laid the matter to rest. Although it is unlikely that any chemistry is involved, the Royal Society of Chemistry in 2012 announced a competition to find 'the best and most creative explanation of the phenomenon' (the correct one would be better, I feel). Twenty-two thousand entries came in. The answer is still not known.

6
Tolerance

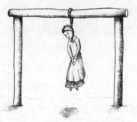

'I feele not in my selfe those common antipathies'

Religio Medici

I N EARLY 2014, anti-Semitism is on the rise across Europe. Islamo-phobia – a word that barely existed until the 1990s – is widespread. In London, the Metropolitan Police stands charged, permanently it seems, with 'institutional racism', a situation doubtless reflected in other cities, and doubtless reflective to some unplumbed extent of the feelings of the majority of the people they protect. Our views about 'travellers', migrants and asylum seekers are formed in ignorance and suspicion.

But we have surely made progress since the seventeenth century.

Norwich's greatest failure of tolerance may be this. In Holy Week of 1144, according to a hagiography produced soon afterwards by a monk newly arrived in the city, a twelve-year-old boy called William was lured away from home with the promise of work and then ritually tortured and crucified by Jews. His body was found in Thorpe Woods beyond Mousehold Heath with a wooden teasel stuffed into the mouth.

Norwich did not at first rise against its Jewish population – a small community had settled in the shadow of the Norman castle, on the site where Thomas Browne's house would later be built. It was only later, possibly when the Church saw an opportunity to create a cult around the 'martyr' William, who is depicted in various East Anglian rood screens with thorns piercing his head and bearing his own cross, that the story grew into the first medieval accusation of blood libel against the Jews, and the pogroms began. In 2004, as work was beginning on the construction of a new shopping centre in the city, seventeen skeletons, including those of eleven children, were discovered at the bottom of an old well. DNA tests proved inconclusive (religion is not genetic). But other evidence strongly supported the theory that the remains were those of Jews slaughtered some time after about 1150.

Following increasing persecution, England's Jews were expelled in 1290. It was not until 1655 that they were readmitted and a small Sephardic community was established in London. Thomas Browne therefore knew no Jews in Norwich, and nor did almost everybody else in England. People nevertheless believe, as Browne states it in *Pseudodoxia Epidemica*, 'That the *Jews* stink naturally, that is, that in their race and nation there is an evil savour.' This is 'a received opinion we know not how to admit', he adds.

Browne does not follow our contemporary liberal reflex and spontaneously reject this insult outright. Instead, shockingly perhaps, he turns to comparative zoology. It is not unreasonable that men should smell if other animals do, he points out. Nor is it improbable that persons may have individual odours detectable, if not by their fellows, then at least by their dogs (Alexander the Great smelt especially delicious, according to Theophrastus). This comparison with animals may serve as a reminder of how lowly many Christians regarded Jews (even if they never met one), but for Browne it is a habitual dimension of his scientific enquiry. Now he comes to his judgement: 'But that an unsavoury odour is gentilitious or national unto the *Jews*, if rightly understood, we cannot well concede; nor will the information of reason or sence induce it.' Browne's use of the word 'gentilitious' is a clear signal that the imputation of malodorousness might also be made, with equal unfairness, against any non-Jewish nation. Browne's own mongrel theory is that Jewishness, 'however pretended to be pure, must needs have suffered inseparated commixtures with nations of all sorts'. This in fact squares well with modern genetic studies which show that there is often little to distinguish Jewish people from many non-Jewish Levantines.

Browne's determination to explore this topic in all scientific earnestness next leads him to examine possible links between diet and human odour. If anything, he argues, Jews should be less odorous than the rest of the population – and indeed healthier – because of their dietary laws, which proscribe the eating of too much meat and other excesses, and hence 'prevent generation of crudities'.

Logic is on his side too. Though they are 'of the same seed', converted Jews are never accused of exuding this odour. It is 'as though Aromatized by their conversion, they lost their scent with their Religion,' he notes. Some people in the seventeenth century suspect that Jews go among them, hiding their true religion; but if that were the case surely then 'could they be smelled out'.

Finally, Browne brings in personal testimony. There may be no Jews in Norwich, but he has certainly met Jews in Padua where there was a ghetto much like the one in nearby Venice. In both Padua and Leiden, Jews were able to enroll as students, often studying medicine. In conversation with them, and even entering the synagogue, he can recall no smell. The origin of the popular slur he traces ultimately to a biblical metaphor of abomination being taken as literal. He ends with some wisdom that modern xenophobes would do well to remember, 'it being a dangerous point to annex a constant property unto any Nation'.

Browne is more critical of Islam: 'the Alcoran of the Turks (I speake without prejudice) is an ill composed Piece, containing in it vaine and ridiculous errours in Philosophy, impossibilities, fictions, and vanities beyond laughter,' he asserts confidently in *Religio Medici*. That parenthetical phrase may read to us now a bit like 'I'm not racist but…', yet he does truly endeavour to speak without prejudice, for his thoughts often lead him to comparisons with more familiar Christian texts where he also finds plenty that is ridiculous.

He does not itemize the vanities of the Qur'an. Browne's chief regret is the squandering of Arab scholarship occasioned by the spread of this religious text, and the ensuing 'policy of Ignorance, deposition of Universities, and banishment of Learning, that hath gotten foot by armes and violence'. His own religion is of course hardly blameless in this regard, and he compares the Muslims' abolition of universities with the Christian propensity to condemn literature, which he suggests arises again from over-literal interpretation of scripture, in this case the injunction, 'Beware lest any man spoil you through philosophy', contained in Saint Paul's letter to the Colossians.

Being closer to the events, scholars in the seventeenth century were in some ways more aware than they are today of the great debt that the Western Renaissance owed to Arab intellectuals. These men preserved the science of the ancient Greek and Roman world, and built substantially on it, especially in the fields of mathematics, medicine, astronomy and chemistry. Browne singles out the alchemist Geber (Jābir ibn Hayyān), who developed the theory that all metals were composed of different proportions of mercury and sulphur, and Avicenna (Ibn Sīnā), the author of medical textbooks used up until medieval times. Such thinkers could surely never be satisfied with the Prophet Muhammad's explanation of earthquakes as 'the motion of a great Bull, upon whose horns all earth is poised'. With examples like this, 'is it not without wonder, how those learned Arabicks so tamely delivered up their belief unto the absurdities of the Alcoran'.

Browne nevertheless sees it as his duty to enlighten readers of *Pseudodoxia Epidemica* as to some of the curious aspects of Muslim worship. In a long discussion of the deceptive nature of east and west (deceptive at least to those who believe the Earth is round because the two must meet), he mentions their holy cities, Mecca and Medina, the places where the Prophet was born and is buried. Although Muslims in the west face east when they pray, in order to face Mecca, Muslims in the east must face west, he points out. The ceremonial is only 'Topical'; there is no mystery or magic in it. Furthermore, he refutes the idea that

Muhammad's tomb in Medina hangs, as some have said, suspended in the air without support – even with the aid of magnets. The 'conceit is fabulous and evidently false from the testimony of Ocular Testators, who affirm his Tomb is made of Stone, and lyeth upon the ground'.

Demystifications such as these are an important feature of Browne's discussion of religions about which most people know little and fear much. They are something we need again today, with media scares about 'unlabelled' halal meat and the insinuation of elements of sharia law into Western legal practice.

Colour was a mystery in the seventeenth century. Why is grass green? Why do other plants have white roots and black seeds, or yellow roots and purple flowers? Why can the fashionable tulip be cultivated to produce almost every colour except blue? When the chemical nature of pigments lay undiscovered, there was no way to begin to explore the matter. Browne asks the questions – and makes a fair attempt to answer them, proposing that colours are due to particular mixtures of the elements. (He means the four ancient elements, not the modern chemical elements, but he is right in principle, as it is often the presence of particular elements, such as magnesium in chlorophyll or iron in haem, that alters the colour of otherwise chemically similar substances.)

Browne is warming up to his real topic, which is 'Of the Blackness of *Negroes*', to which he devotes two substantial chapters and a further digression in *Pseudodoxia Epidemica*. He wants to answer the question of 'Why some men, yea and they a mighty and considerable part of mankind, should first acquire and still retain the gloss and tincture of blackness?' His exploration follows the usual rambling path, discounting fanciful theories based on causes ranging from the natural to the mythological, and diverting into the coloration of animals in different latitudes. Unlike the stoat or the mountain hare, Browne notes, dark-skinned people transplanted into Europe's 'cold and flegmatick habitations' do not turn white. Nor are their children born paler than they. Unless they mix with people of paler complexion, that is: Browne is relaxed about racial mixing, as are many at this time. The first anti-miscegenation laws were only introduced in 1664 in the American colonies, when Maryland outlawed marriage between white people and slaves. The prohibition was soon extended to any marriage between races and was not overturned in many southern states until 1967.

Browne eliminates 'the fervour of the Sun' as the primary cause of blackness, pointing out that there are no 'black' people indigenous to the Americas, which span the equator. He concludes instead that the black complexion is exclusively African in origin, there being people in Africa living far from the equator who are as black as any. But as for what produced the original colour 'mutation' – he uncannily uses this word so suggestive of Darwin and modern genetics – this remains 'a Riddle'.

Browne is more interested in the emerging politics of race. He dismisses the opinion that black skin was a curse of God by means of hermeneutical analysis, and with a startlingly modern gust of righteous liberalism: 'Whereas men affirm this colour was a Curse, I cannot make out the propriety of that name, it neither seeming so to them, nor reasonably unto us.' It is simply *difference* that provokes prejudice. He goes much further, finding no reason why black people should not be considered beautiful, the bodily ideal of the Greeks and Romans being all about proportion and saying nothing about colour. (The days when the proportions of various parts of the body would be used – by European 'scientists' – to devise racial hierarchies lay a few decades in the future.) Browne's writing here soars to a meditation on beauty. It is almost as if he has fallen for some negress, as he echoes lines in Shakespeare's 'dark lady' sonnets: 'Then will I sweare beauty her selfe is blacke, / And all they foule that thy complexion lacke.'

Although Browne does not comment on the iniquities of the slave trade, his scientific and moral belief in the unity of humankind is apparent. Long before the European colonial project has reached its peak, he displays a vivid postcolonial imagination, which shows most clearly in the unlikely medium of a spoof verse written in reply to a friend who has sent him a prophecy. Browne responds with his own

'Prophecy Concerning the future state of several Nations', written, like the famous *Prophecies* of Nostradamus, published a century earlier, in rhyme.

Satirically meant or not, I would be disappointed if I did not find that Browne's predictions are a cut above most of those doing the rounds. The verse reads:

When *New England* shall trouble *New Spain*.
When *Jamaica* shall be Lady of the Isles and the Main.
When *Spain* shall be in *America* hid,
And *Mexico* shall prove a *Madrid*.
When *Mahomet*'s Ships on the *Baltick* shall ride,
And Turks shall labour to have Ports on that side,
When *Africa* shall no more sell out their Blacks
To make Slaves and Drudges to the American Tracts.
When *Batavia* the Old shall be contemn'd by the New.
When a new Drove of Tartars shall China subdue.
When *America* shall cease to send out its Treasure,
But employ it at home in American Pleasure.
When the new World shall the old invade,
Nor count them Lords but their fellows in Trade.
When Men shall almost pass to *Venice* by Land,
Not in deep Water but from Sand to Sand.
When *Nova Zembla* shall be no stay
Unto those who pass to or from *Cathay*.
Then think strange things are come to light,
Where but few have had a foresight.

Browne provides his unknown friend with a detailed exegesis of his prophecy that need not concern us here. The predictions are remarkable enough as they stand: the development of African nations, the rise of an Hispanic population in America, the growth of American spending power, the economic expansion of Mexico, and even a Wallander-style fear of Islamists insurgent in Scandinavia. Applying a proper Brownean scepticism, I am bound to add, though, that I see little sign of Tartars subduing China or of the Venetian lagoon silting up.

This embrace of other races and religions stems from one simple thought. In *Religio Medici* Browne writes: 'I hold there is a generall beauty in the works of God, and therefore no deformity in any kind or species of creature whatsoever.' Taking in man as part of creation, as he always does, Browne counts all humankind as formed in equal perfection.

It is Browne's continental tour of the 1630s that has taught him not to fear difference. He is proud – inordinately so, it seems to us now – that foreign foods agree with him; he has shared frogs and snails with the French and, if he is to be believed, locusts with Jews. He points out – and he believes he is new in doing this – the dangerous temptation to stereotype national behaviour and stoutly resists it.

His travels must have tested his mettle. France provided the first real taste of Catholicism for an Englishman born in the year of the Gunpowder Plot. The French Wars of Religion between Catholics and Protestants (1562–1598), ending with the Edict of Nantes safeguarding the rights of Protestants, were still fresh in the memory. Things were especially tense in Montpellier, where Browne studied; having declared itself Huguenot, the city heroically resisted a siege by the king's army in 1622. Padua placed Browne closer to the centre of Catholicism, but in a city and university under the sway of the Venetian republic, where papal dogma came second to commercial and intellectual freedoms. When he travelled north from Italy to Leiden, he would have been made aware once again of religious tensions, this time between the Catholic Spanish Netherlands and the Protestant Dutch Republic. In short, he has passed through 'many reformations; each Countrey proceeding in a particular way and Method...some angrily...others calmely'.

Browne saw rather less of the civil wars that awaited in his own country. The first battles broke out in 1642, not long after he had settled in Norwich. Though East Anglia was largely Parliamentarian (Oliver Cromwell was Member of Parliament for Cambridge) and Browne was by inclination a Royalist, any conflict in Browne's mind was never fully realized on the streets. Though there were intermittent riots protesting against taxes levied by the Parliamentarian forces, the major moment of violence visited upon the city was in fact an accident. On 24 April 1648, there occurred the 'Great Blow', in which the county arms store and ninety-eight barrels of gunpowder were set off in a vast explosion which killed forty people, blew out the windows of St Peter Mancroft church, and rained debris over the marketplace close to where Browne's house stood.

'You might read every word of Sir Thomas Browne's writings and never discover that a sword had been unsheathed or a shot fired in England all the time he was living and writing there,' noted the Scottish preacher Alexander Whyte in his 1898 appreciation of *Religio Medici*. My feeling is that Browne's experience of the English Civil War is a bit like that of Frédéric Moreau in Flaubert's *Sentimental Education*, who misses the revolution of 1848, so wrapped up is he in his own affairs, or like Christopher Lloyd in Julian Barnes's *Metroland*, who follows in his footsteps oblivious of the Paris *événements* of 1968 – or, if I might add my own modest moment of suspended reality, driving home from eating out in central London on the night of the Poll Tax Riots in 1990, vaguely wondering why there were burning cars lying upturned in the roadway.

Whyte's evaluation is not quite accurate, however. There are intriguing hints here and there in Browne's writing that all is not at peace, from a strange preoccupation with Roman battle formations in *The Garden of Cyrus* to the stork we met earlier, said to be found only in republics, a story concocted 'to disparage Monarchical government', he says. Though Browne was a loyal supporter of the king, he was, of course, not unreasoning in his support, and there are times when his thinking appears to align more closely with the Parliamentarian view. In *Pseudodoxia Epidemica*, for example, he writes concerning sources of error that states have no right to deceive the people. The gesture behind publication of this book is also profoundly populist: it could never be perceived, as the work of the Royal Society, founded upon the Restoration of Charles II, perhaps could be, as a means of crown institutions gaining control over new knowledge. Browne 'deprecated the frown of Theology' as Edmund Gosse puts it, meaning that he was no Puritan. But after the Restoration he was, in his private correspondence, nevertheless critical of the king for not reining in his extravagant lifestyle. In all, he walked a careful line.

Browne may suffer from terminal indecision, but its dividend is his almost boundless tolerance for the individual. His attitude towards other religions and races, shaped by his European travels and wide learning, is mostly exemplary; it stands up well to scrutiny today. By the standard of his day, it is almost miraculous in its benevolence. He speaks up for classes of humanity that were often ostracized or demonized. He would have something to add to our current debate on multiculturalism.

He will engage with anybody with whom he can reason. His personal challenge is the multitude, 'that numerous piece of monstrosity, which taken asunder seem men, and the reasonable creatures of God; but confused together, make but one great beast'. This is not a matter of social class, for 'there is a rabble even amongst the Gentry'. It is purely a matter of numbers. It is what the Victorian writer Charles Mackay would call 'the madness of crowds' that baffles him. He would, therefore, like to think of himself as especially wary when weighing the passions of the masses.

But this paragon of tolerance is about to disappoint us. For there is the matter of the witch trial. The story has all the right paraphernalia for a supernatural tale. It involves unappealing old women, innocent children driven into fits and swoons, props including vomited pins, extra nipples and a toad, and an untimely death. Or, to put it another way, it involves feared women on the margins of society, comfortable accusers with manufactured grievances, class friction, hallucinations and delusions, ignorance and credulousness, and the misfortune of sudden illness with no apparent natural cause or cure.

On 10 March 1662, two widows from Lowestoft were brought before the assizes at Bury St Edmunds in Suffolk. They had been charged the year before with bewitching seven children and young women of the town. Rose Cullender was probably about sixty years old at the time of the trial and had been widowed for twenty-three years. But she was not poor, like many accused witches, and she lived in the house which had passed to her son when her husband died. Amy Denny, or Duny, was rather younger and was more recently widowed. It is likely that her husband had been a persistent minor criminal in the Lowestoft area. She lived in rented accommodation on the southern fringe of the town.

The two women's interactions with their accusers were commercial before they came to be seen as supernatural. Amy Denny was called upon for ad hoc childcare duties, and both of the women had sought to buy herring from two of the plantiffs' houses. The first of these exchanges had occurred five years to the day before the trial began, the others intermittently thereafter.

The first to testify was Dorothy Durrant, a tradesman's wife. On 10 March 1657, she told the court, she had asked Amy Denny to look after her infant son, William, for a short period while she attended to some business away from home. William was just twenty months old, and Dorothy stressed that Denny was not to suckle him. When Dorothy returned, Denny apparently explained that she had offered the infant her breast. After a row, she left the house in high dudgeon. That night, the boy fell into 'swounding' that lasted for several weeks. Dorothy then called a Yarmouth doctor known for treating bewitched children. The witch-doctor advised her to hang up the infant's blanket during the day in order to shake out anything that might be in it, which should then be burnt. When this was done, a large toad fell out and was caught and thrown onto the fire, where it exploded with a loud pop. William recovered following this, while Amy Denny was found the next day with scorch marks over her face, making further curses against the Durrant family.

A couple of years later, Dorothy's elder stepdaughter, Elizabeth, then aged about ten, complained of being afflicted by Denny. When Dorothy returned from the apothecary where she had gone to get medicine for Elizabeth, she found Amy Denny in her home, paying an unbidden visit to the sick child. Denny departed, saying the child would not live long. Elizabeth died two days later, while Dorothy became so lame in her legs that she required crutches.

The next witness was Samuel Pacy, a well-to-do fish merchant, the father of Elizabeth and Deborah, respectively about twelve and eight years of age. The prime mover behind the charges, Pacy had had Amy Denny put in the stocks as punishment for a first offence of witchcraft the previous year. Now he described how the sickly Deborah was one day taken lame. When Denny came to the house to buy herring a week later, she was repeatedly turned away. Upon being sent away for a third time, Denny grumbled something and Deborah, seeing this, was taken with severe fits. After this, their father told the court, both sisters began to experience **hallucinations** of Amy Denny and also Rose Cullender, and fell into fits and swoons. Between them they vomited up more than forty crooked pins as well as a 'twopenny nail with a very broad head', which were produced as evidence in court.

Elizabeth was present in the court, but apparently unable to speak or move during the proceedings, except for one remarkable episode which

❧⁓❧⁓❧⁓❧⁓❧⁓❧⁓❧⁓❧ ❧⁓ ❧⁓ ❧⁓❧⁓❧⁓❧⁓❧⁓❧⁓❧⁓❧

hallucination (PE, 1646): Browne defines hallucination as occurring if vision be 'depraved and receive its objects erroneously'. He implies that the word is in current usage with this meaning, and does not claim to invent it (although Browne's usage is the earliest citation given in the OED). This corresponds well with modern definitions such as Webster's: 'perception of objects with no reality usu. arising from disorder of the nervous system or in response to drugs (as LSD)'. Were unicorns, basilisks or witches hallucinations? Browne did not believe so. They were all subject to rational explanation. Were the apparitions described by bewitched children hallucinations? By his own definition, Browne should have thought them so. But no; they were understood as appearances of reality – solid enough to be admissible in court as 'spectral evidence', as they were at Bury, and as similar apparitions would be later at Salem, and impossible to refute. According to Carl Sagan, it was not until the eighteenth century that the role of hallucinations in the persecution of witches began to be properly recognized.

took place away from the main trial, as we shall see. Deborah was in such a bad state that her parents did not even bring her to the assizes. But the girls' failure to testify for themselves was more than compensated for by Samuel's evidence, which was copious and lurid in its detail and delivered in a sober manner that greatly impressed the court officials.

Sixteen-year-old Jane Bocking was also too weak to attend court, but her mother Diana testified that she had experienced fits and stomach pains and had vomited up pins, accusing both Denny and Cullender. Edmund Durrant (apparently unrelated to the other Durrants) testified that Rose Cullender had come to his house to buy herrings, but when she was sent away empty-handed, she afflicted his daughter Ann with the same symptoms. Ann was silent in court but fell into renewed fits when brought before the accused. Susan Chandler, eighteen years old and employed in service in Lowestoft, was likewise silent at the trial. Her mother Mary described the same symptoms and also accused Cullender. Mary Chandler had been one of six townswomen appointed to strip-search Cullender at the time the arrest warrant was issued. They had found first one 'thing like a teat' on her lower belly, then others 'in her privy parts'. It was following this that Cullender had bewitched her daughter. Ann Baldinge, a single woman aged seventeen years, testified that Cullender had bewitched her too, just a few weeks before the assizes. Other accusers included further family members, various town officials, and Cullender's landlady.

The judge was Sir Matthew Hale, one of the most senior judges in England, known for his humane and fair-minded treatment of prisoners in his dock. Though broadly a Royalist, he was notably lenient in cases where national security was supposedly under threat, and portrayed himself in his memoirs as a champion of the oppressed. But he had tried witchcraft cases before and passed the death penalty.

I cannot relate the full details of the trial, which lasted four days. The story is superbly told and analysed by Gilbert Geis, an emeritus professor of criminology at the University of California, and Ivan Bunn, a local historian in Suffolk, in their book *A Trial of Witches*. The book also includes in an appendix the only first-hand account of the court proceedings, though this was first published as late as 1682, some twenty years after the events it describes, by an anonymous agent, who claims in a preface to have come by the original transcript of the court proceedings 'in a private gentleman's hands in the country'. The document has been shown to be unreliable, with discrepancies between the manuscript and printed versions. It even wrongly dates the trial to 1664.

It is time to call forth our expert. It is not clear why Thomas Browne was present at the Bury assize, but it is probable that he was summoned by those seeking to secure a conviction of the accused women. He had tenuous social connections with at least one of the court officials and with the principal plaintiff, Samuel Pacy.

He makes his entry at a key juncture. After the plaintiff families have all given their evidence, the proceedings are unexpectedly interrupted by 'divers known persons', according to the 1682 record. These are three serjeants-at-law – officers with duties of arrest and enforcing

A

TRYAL

OF

WITCHES,

AT THE

ASSIZES

HELD AT

Bury St. Edmonds for the County of *SUFFOLK*; on the Tenth day of *March*, 1664.

BEFORE

Sir MATTHEW HALE Kt.

THEN

Lord Chief Baron of His Majesties Court of EXCHEQUER.

Taken by a Person then Attending the Court

LONDON,
Printed for *William Shrewsbery* at the Bible in *Duck-Lane*. 1682.

judgement – who are unhappy about the prospect of a conviction based on 'the imagination only of the parties afflicted'. (The unease of all three was redacted in the record to name only one doubter among them, John Keeling.) Two modern-seeming measures might serve to demonstrate proper impartiality: an independent expert witness; and an experimental test.

The testimony of 'Dr. *Brown* of *Norwich*, a Person of great knowledge', in the words of the 1682 report, is brief. He gives his view that the 'afflicted persons' were truly bewitched. This is a matter of simple medical opinion, presumably based on observing their erratic behaviour in the courtroom. He then expands on this, recalling a recent case he has heard of in Denmark where witches had been discovered using the very same method of affliction by pins and nails. Such 'swounding fits were natural, and nothing else but that they call them other',* Browne suggests, 'heightened to a great excess by the subtilty of the devil, cooperating with the malice of these which we term witches, at whose instance he doth these villanies'. It is a fine distinction indeed that he draws between natural illness and supernatural affliction.

This is the sum of Browne's contribution according to the court record. He may or may not have been present for the remainder of the trial. It is a loss if he was not, since it involves an experiment whose conduct and outcome should have greatly interested him.

The reason for going to the further trouble of an experiment to determine the guilt or innocence of the accused may lie with the judge himself. For Matthew Hale was a man who recognized the value of empirical observation in the testing of hypotheses. In 1674, he would publish an account of his own scientific investigation, *Difficiles Nugae: Or, Observations Touching the Torricellian Experiment, and The various Solutions of the same, especially touching the Weight and Elasticity of the AIR.* (The

---

* The transcript here reads, '…but that they call the Mother', but sense seems to indicate it is 'them other' that is meant, in other words that the afflicted persons ascribe *supernatural* causes to their illness. There again, 'mother' was at the time a colloquial synonym for the uterus and for hysteria. (Nick Rennison)

publisher was the same as for the trial report.) Torricelli's famous experiment demonstrated the existence of barometric pressure by inverting a tube containing mercury, sealed at one end, over a bath of mercury; when this is done, the mercury in the tube falls to a leave behind a pure vacuum above it that is a standard length of about 76 centimetres. Hale could not believe that this volume was an empty void. He believed that in God's creation everything was suspended from the sky and thus that there was no requirement for the atmosphere to exert such a downward pressure. More broadly, he felt that scientists, once in possession of an exciting theory, have a way of losing their impartiality when it comes to considering challenging new evidence. Torricelli thought he had a vacuum, but others had repeated the experiment and reached different conclusions. Could Hale disprove him once and for all?

How is this science at all connected with witchcraft? To Hale, the concept of a vacuum – nothing – implies that everywhere else is occupied by something, by matter, and this leaves no space for the spiritual. If there are regions where the Holy Spirit does not reach, then this may be where the devil and his witches reign. Hale replicates Torricelli's apparatus and discovers, when he puts his finger over the end of the glass tube, a force of attraction sucking on his fingertip. 'Most evidently the force that the finger feels is from within, and not from without,' he writes, suggesting that it is not, as Torricelli believes, air pressure all around that is producing the sensation. For Hale, there had to be a physical something in the void responsible for the attraction. 'First therefore I say it is not Nothing, or a pure Vacuity, but it is some corporeal substance that succeeds in the head of the Tube, derelicted by the Mercury.'

The experiment conducted in the Bury courtrooms was very different, although just as scientific in its way. In the first instance, the accused women were instructed to touch the afflicted girls 'in the midst of their Fitts'. Only they, it was found, had the (demonic) power to release them. Next, the girls were made to place their aprons over their heads so they could not see. Rose Cullender was then instructed to touch them, which produced the same change as before. At this, however, an 'ingenious person' in the court objected that the girls might still be counterfeiting. The court officials then resolved on a more careful experiment. This time, in a private part of the court building, before a select few observers, one of the girls was again blinded with her apron, and one of the accused, this time Amy Denny, brought forward. But instead of her being made to carry on and touch the girl as before, another person stepped in to do this, 'which produced the same effect as the touch of the Witch did in the Court'. This simple substitution should of course have been enough to show that a conviction would be unsafe. Surely now the girl *had* to be confeiting. But the witnesses returned to the court more confused than ever, protesting that they must have seen some kind of imposture, and the judge was unconvinced.

Would this little drama have altered Browne's opinion? Probably, it would have confirmed it, making the children's affliction seem less organic, and more maleficent.

The trial now moved toward its end. The judge did not sum up the case for the jury, lest, as he explained, he introduce his own bias. But he told them the questions they had to answer: were the children bewitched, and were the accused women guilty of the bewitching? Browne had affirmed that the former was the case, but had apparently said nothing specifically to implicate the women in the dock. But once bewitchment was agreed, who else was there to blame? The sentence was passed and the abbreviation *sus per coll* inked into the original indictments – *suspendendae per collum*, to be hanged by the neck. Verdict given, most of the girls made a spontaneous recovery; Dorothy Durrant walked again. Amy Denny and Rose Cullender were hanged on 17 March. The last words in the trial record: 'but they confessed nothing'.

Where does the Bury trial sit on the historical timeline of English witchcraft? Was witchcraft on the rise or on its way out? Were the proceedings a fair example of modern jurisprudence or a throwback to more superstitious times? We need to know if we are to understand Browne's testimony and certainly if we are hoping to excuse his actions.

A belief in witches and evil magic is of course as old as Eden, but the practice of witchcraft was only made a capital offence in England in 1542. The witchcraft act in use at the time of the Bury trial was passed in 1604, the year after the accession to the English throne of James I, and was influenced by his exploration of the topic in his book *Daemonologie*. This law remained on the statute book until 1736, but the last woman to be judicially hanged as a witch in England went to her death well before this, in 1685, although there were occasional vigilante lynchings until well into the nineteenth century.

The Bury trial thus falls somewhere after the peak of the English witch frenzy, which gathered momentum in the 1560s, and included the notorious episode of the Pendle witches in 1612 and the activities of the 'witch-finder general', Matthew Hopkins, chiefly in Essex and Suffolk during the 1640s. In 1645, Hopkins had chosen Bury St Edmunds as the site of a special court (properly constituted courts being hard to convene during the Civil War) at which eighteen 'witches' were hanged. In all, Hopkins's campaign accounted for almost half of the estimated 500 people ever executed for witchcraft in England. It is notable that legal action against witches spiked at times of national tension, such as in the 1580s, when there were fears of invasion and regicide, and during the Civil War years. With the Restoration in 1660, relative normality is regained.

The trial of 1662 nevertheless casts a long shadow that reaches across the Atlantic to the infamous Salem witch trials thirty years later – trials that, according to Geis and Bunn, 'might not have taken place if there had not been a trial at Bury St. Edmunds'. Their reason for this startling claim is that the movers behind the Salem trials, including the Massachusetts Puritan minister Cotton Mather, believing that 'witchcrafts here most exactly resemble the witchcrafts there', wished to proceed in proper fashion, and took the 1682 account of the Bury trial as their guide.

In parallel with this crisp timeline of historical events there is another, fuzzier line which shows that witchcraft did not simply rise and fall during the course of the seventeenth century, but that at all times it was a matter of dispute and uncertainty, even though it had a certain status in law.

There were of course those who firmly believed in witches throughout this period. Thomas Browne has to be counted as one of these. 'I have ever beleeved, and doe now know, that there are Witches,' he writes in *Religio Medici*. He has hardly shifted his position by the sixth edition of *Pseudodoxia Epidemica* thirty years later, where he writes of the devil as an agent of error whose devious methods include 'endeavours to propagate the unbelief of Witches'. For him, belief in witches is a theological necessity: belief in God entails a belief also in the devil, and belief in the devil means belief also in his agents, witches and demons. Those who deny the existence of witches can only be atheists in this view. Contemporaries such as the religious scholar Méric Casaubon pursued a more nuanced line, admitting certain natural explanations for witchcraft, including medical explanations, while still upholding belief in witches themselves, fearing that denial would encourage atheism.

But there were sceptics. Oddly, one Dr Browne, a physician of Norwich, was in 1578 accused of spreading mistrust in the law by asserting that witches did not exist. Even some of those inclined to go along with the law and Christian doctrine could see that it was hard to say exactly who was a witch. The arts of sorcery could be acquired through academic study, for example, as well as from the devil, which meant that not all those who cast spells were true witches. Contrary to popular belief, witch trials in fact often led to acquittals (except where zealots like Hopkins were running proceedings). In later trials, doubts began to be raised about the reliability of witnesses. In 1675, eight Stockholm women were accused of witchcraft by a number of children, including some of their own. But the children's testimony that they had been carried off to a witches' sabbath was shown to be unreliable when their stories did not agree. Some of the children who refused to cease their accusations were sentenced to death to stop the stories spreading, and some of the accused women were released.

More forthright opinions began to be voiced. The Yorkshire physician and occultist John Webster wrote *The Displaying of Supposed Witchcraft* in 1677, in which he argued that witches did not exist and that belief in them only arose from mistranslations in the Bible. His view was endorsed by the Royal Society, though not, unsurprisingly, by the Church. Joseph Glanvill, an early fellow of the Royal Society, positioned himself as a sceptic's sceptic, keen to take witchcraft at face value as a legitimate topic for scientific investigation. There were soon so many eager debunkers of witchcraft that even people who should have disbelieved, such as the scientist Robert Boyle, felt driven to affirm its existence. The sceptics themselves stood to be demonized along with the witches. Witchcraft was thus still widely believed and accepted during the rest of Browne's life. Thereafter, witches began to be seen as harmless; by 1750 in Norwich it was 'no offence to be a Witch but to pretend to be so which is very penall'.

'The Bury trial is interesting for the light it throws on how a witch trial could be conducted after the Restoration (especially in Bury, site of the notorious Hopkins trials in 1645),' according to the historian Ian Bostridge. It was 'a model witch trial'. The doubts aired, experiments conducted, and independent opinion heard all contributed to this impression. Browne fills the role of the expert whom Casaubon recommends should be present at witch trials. He 'makes the necessary discrimination between natural and supernatural'. He explains that bewitching is the act of the devil, aided by witches. But he does not say that the accused women *are* witches. There again, he doesn't say they are not, or apparently propose any better way of testing the matter.

Seventeenth-century justice has been done. The twenty-first century stands dismayed. Model it may be, but the Bury trial stands as an illustration to us now of the dangers of letting Christian doctrine dictate the actions of English courts, or any religion dictate any judicial proceeding. It also shows that those who go about with the assurance that they are rational beings using the latest scientific methods can still lead us into dark corners.

Can we exonerate Browne? Even to explain his actions, we need to see the events described and enacted in court not in the self-congratulatory terms of our own supposed enlightenment but in terms of his own century. We know that a toad could easily have tumbled out of a blanket in a dank house, although we know too that toads are popularly associated with witchcraft, and the image of a toad, once suggested, would be hard for people to get out of their heads. We know that the vomited pins and nails produced in court, another entirely standard feature of such cases, could easily be faked, but we know too that swallowing objects is a classic behaviour observed in people with certain mental disorders. We know that the extraneous teats are probably hernias or some other organic growth. We know that the women's behaviour – grumbling and cursing when they do not get what they have come for – is perhaps no more than the habitual resentment of those made to feel socially inferior.

Why can't the rationalist in Browne see this? Because he sees something else first. Like Hale and others in the courtroom, he sees evidence of his Christian faith in the existence of witchcraft and witches. There is also a secular reason guiding Browne. Thinkers such as Hobbes and Casaubon understood that witchcraft is an imagined activity, but one that should nevertheless continue to be called criminal in order to bind Church and state authority together. A guilty verdict at Bury, so soon after the Restoration, will act as a social glue, enabling all religious factions to unite against a common evil.

In a modern play of Browne's life, the witch trial would undoubtedly be the pivotal scene after which nothing is the same again. But there is every sign that it was no such moment. Browne carried on regardless. He never wrote about the trial, his role in it, or the fate of the accused women. In his commonplace book some years after the trial, there is only this: 'Wee are no way doubtfull that there are wiches, butt have not been alwayes satisfied in the application of their wichcrafts or whether parties accused or suffering have been guiltie of that abomination.' Is this a specific regret, or Browne's customary hedging generalized to cover all eventualities?

A few weeks after I met Kevin Faulkner, the Browne enthusiast, he sends me an email. It seems I have not allayed his fears about how I might represent Browne. 'I am not totally sure whether my interest in

Browne will be portrayed in a very favourable light in any forthcoming publication of yours,' he writes. 'Like all good scientists, including Browne, you have a strong grain of scepticism about him. Not sure that judging him from the vantage-point of our age always the wisest. Too easy to condemn him without any empathy or full understanding of the intellectual climate of his age which shifted considerably in his lifetime. If you look closely the same fixed viewpoints in *Religio Medici* are reiterated by him in old age. What do you think?'

Who might be the victims of 'witch-hunts' and 'witch trials' today? The terms are bandied about by those with a sharp sense of grievance. Bankers in New York and London have claimed they were the victims of a witch-hunt when proposals were brought in to limit their bonuses following the financial crisis of 2008. An ally of Lord Rennard, the former chief executive of the Liberal Democrats accused of groping female parliamentary candidates, has compared his friend's treatment by the party's leadership to the Salem witch trials.

But these are absurd examples. We need to establish some firmer parameters. First, for the experience of the twenty-first-century accused to be at all comparable to that of the seventeenth-century 'witch', there must be an element of public mania leading up to the arraignment or apparent during the judicial process. Second, the case is likely to involve a plaintiff and defendant who are known to each other, or who are participants in some unequal social transaction. Third, we should have a sense that the alleged crime is something that in other places or in future times might be understood in more enlightened ways.

Paedophiles seem an obvious group to start with. Those who are guilty truly do horrible things and great harm to children, of course, but the blind frenzy of hate that surrounds our fears means it is easy to accuse the innocent. Social workers deemed to have been negligent or worse in their duties are perhaps a closer fit. They are often women, have a duty of care of children who are not their own, and are seen by some to exert 'unreasonable' powers. Their unfavourable judgement of our parenting abilities may seem not unlike a curse, and they are able in a final resort to 'take' our children. There are websites where you can 'name and shame' people you suspect to be in either group.

The parallel with witch trials is not exact in either case, because we know witches do not exist. But there still seems to be something about the way society treats both groups that reaches back through the centuries. I share my quandary with a barrister friend who isolates the difficulty I am having: 'These days, we tend not to try people if they've not done anything,' he says drily. He's right, of course. But it occurs to me that his statement might equally well have been made by any seventeenth-century prosecutor. We only try people for the crimes of the day.

Let us expand our search. There is no shortage of contemporary cases that have an air of moral panic about them. One of the most notorious of recent years is that of Amanda Knox, accused together with Raffaele Sollecito of the murder of a fellow student, Meredith Kercher, in Perugia, Italy, in 2007. Knox claims to have been called *strega* – witch – by lawyers representing the man she falsely named under police questioning as the perpetrator. Vocal, pretty, and erratic in her behaviour, Knox became the focus of intense media speculation. This was sustained throughout the original trial, the subsequent appeal and a retrial. Following the guilty verdict reinstated at the retrial, Knox has continued to protest her innocence in very public ways, for example posting online a picture of herself holding a placard in Italian proclaiming her innocence. This produced a backlash in Italy, but as Knox herself has observed: 'Whether they mean to or not, these *Perugia vi odia* ['Perugia hates you'] people, who bear their emotions on placards, are helping me and the world to understand what has really happened in this case.'

Italian sisters Elisabetta and Francesca Grillo had been employed for years as assistants in the household of the cookery writer Nigella Lawson and her then husband, the art collector Charles Saatchi. In 2012, they were accused of using credit cards they had been given for work for their own gain. At a pre-trial hearing, the Grillos reneged on an agreement to conceal Lawson's use of drugs from her husband, and in the trial itself complained of ill treatment at the hands of their employers. The case has the mutual dependence, the grant of trust, and the outsider element of historic witch trials. It soon became apparent that the two accused were merely a lightning rod for Saatchi's and Lawson's marital difficulties. As the marriage imploded, the Grillos were found not guilty, and it was soon Lawson who felt that a 'witch hunt' had been launched against her.

In 2013, Bijan Ebrahimi, a disabled Iranian immigrant, was maliciously identified as a paedophile by neighbours after he was accused of photographing children vandalizing his garden. Police were called, but it was Ebrahimi who found himself arrested, a crowd taunting him as he was driven away. Finding no truth in the accusations, the police then released him. Two days later, he was viciously murdered by the father of the children he had photographed, and his body was burnt. His real crime, in the eyes of his vigilante killer, was presumably his otherness – his foreignness and his disability. The first victim of the witch-finder Matthew Hopkins in 1644 was the one-legged widow Elizabeth Clarke of Manningtree.

A special hatred – driven by incomprehension and the deep fear that we have the capacity to do the same ourselves – is reserved for mothers accused of killing their own children. In 1999, Sally Clark was convicted of the murder of her two infant children in 1996 and 1998 (they were later shown to have died from 'cot death'). The popular press treated her with the brightly coloured vitriol it reserves for 'evil' child killers. But Clark's persecution was worse in prison where, as a solicitor and daughter of a police officer, as well as an apparently unrepentant child killer, she was an easy target. However, it was later shown that the conviction had been based on flawed expert testimony. The paediatrician Sir Roy Meadow had asserted in court that the odds of a single cot death in such a family were 1 in 8,500, and therefore that the odds of two such deaths would be 1 in 73 million (8,500 x 8,500 rounded up) – so unlikely that it was effectively ruled out as a cause of both deaths, as Clark's defence was claiming; double murder was statistically far more likely. In fact, the chances of a double cot death in the same family cannot be calculated in this way. Nevertheless, the jury returned a majority guilty verdict, and Clark served three years in prison before being freed on appeal. Clark never came to terms with the actions of a legal system in which she herself had invested her career, and she was found dead of alcohol poisoning in her home four years later.

Social workers are often the focus of public vilification: the work they do – intervening where normal social structures have failed – is poorly understood and is backed by state powers of control over people's lives. Oversights and errors can have tragic consequences. In 2007, the death of 'Baby P' produced a public outcry against social workers in the London borough of Haringey, where the infant was on an at-risk register because of violent treatment by his mother and others. The ultimate focus of the witch-hunt in this case was not the mother but the borough's head of children's services, Sharon Shoesmith, who, although she had not been directly involved in the decisions in the case, had had the temerity to defend her department and her own position, which made her seem callous in the eyes of the media. The *Sun* newspaper amassed a petition with more than a million signatures calling for 'smug' Shoesmith to go. She was eventually sacked by the government minister with responsibility for children, but later won financial compensation for unfair dismissal. It is argued that many children have been saved as a result of the moral panic in this case, although it also became harder to recruit social workers.

Following the exposure of the well-known disc jockey Jimmy Savile as a paedophile after his death in 2011, a wider enquiry was launched into claims of historical child abuse and sexual exploitation by a number of well-known media figures in Britain. Michael Le Vell was one of three actors in the popular *Coronation Street* television soap opera to be arrested. Le Vell was accused and later acquitted of child abuse offences including rape.* At first the UK Crown Prosecution Service had not

---

* Customary judicial advice to treat rape allegations with extreme scepticism, assiduously followed in many British and American trials until feminist

sought to bring a case, but a review of evidence and fresh allegations – and then the breaking news of Savile's history – led to a reassessment that there would be a 'realistic prospect of conviction'. Two other actors in the series were also cleared of similar offences, and the CPS was then accused of having launched a 'celebrity witch hunt'. These verdicts do not of course prove that prominent persons have not used their celebrity to prey upon impressionable and vulnerable persons, nor do they show that their accusers are malicious fantasists. Nevertheless, it is hard to believe that the pursuit of these investigations with such vigour so long after they were alleged to have happened does not represent some kind of displacement activity away from things we do not want to confront that are happening in our society now.

These modern 'witch trials' reveal what witch trials always have the potential to reveal: the limits of our tolerance and the shape of our own deepest fears and weaknesses. Our human response to such cases may have changed, but perhaps not as much as we like to think. We tell ourselves that we no longer seek out witches, but somehow we still find them brought before us. The courts stand in judgement, appearing harsh in some cases, lenient in others, as they are bound to do if they are society's instrument of fairness. The major difference between now and then is surely the role played by the media, which ensures that our collective reaction has not progressed as far as the individual response of our better nature, and which appoints itself in the Matthew Hopkins role as the chief rooter out of 'evil'.

There have been more extreme examples of moral panic that have the explicit Christian dimension that accusations of witchcraft seem to demand. During the 1980s the United States and then Britain and other countries experienced a wave of 'satanic abuse' cases where social services removed children from pre-school, day-care facilities or their families because they were said to be victims of abuses that included elements

---

campaigning in the 1970s, originates in notes on recommended legal procedure made by Matthew Hale, probably in the 1670s.

of ritual. Tales spread of bestiality, child sacrifice and cannibalism. In Britain, seven children from an extended family were taken into care in Nottinghamshire, twenty were taken into care in Rochdale, nine on the Orkney island of South Ronaldsay, and there were other similar instances. No evidence of ritual abuse was ever found, despite allegations made not only by concerned adults but also by the child victims. In a veritable throwback to the seventeenth century, in some cases lack of evidence was itself cited as evidence of the devilish deviousness of the perpetrators.

Subsequent investigation into the handling of these incidents found that the social workers had been too ready to believe the children's stories and unwilling to take denials of wrongdoing at face value. They had used flawed interviewing techniques in which leading questions and 'anatomically correct' dolls served to project interviewers' imagined versions of what might have happened onto the children's accounts. The apparent clustering of satanic abuses turned out in some cases to be an effect of the way that social services categorized the children – an excess of zeal to echo the statistical blip produced in Essex and Suffolk by the witch-finder Hopkins in 1645, according to Jean La Fontaine, a social anthropologist who examined the modern epidemic.

This is not to say that these satanic abuse claims can be attributed to a wholly irrational mass hysteria, or that nothing depraved was going on. Recently uncovered paedophile rings made more plausible the extrapolation to satanic cults. Many other factors doubtless contributed: the breakdown of nuclear family life, evangelical Christianity, millenarian fears, the spread of violent and sexual imagery on video, and so on. Nor were social workers' fears entirely unfounded; in some cases, children had been encouraged to repeat lurid stories in order to provide a smokescreen that would lead investigators to discredit claims of 'ordinary' abuses. In the end, though, 'satanic' meant little more than 'organized'. As La Fontaine writes in her study, *Speak of the Devil*: 'Mackay regarded the belief in witchcraft as a popular delusion, but 150 years later, social scientists do not dismiss it so lightly.'

Furthermore witchcraft is a living tradition in many countries. Belief in witches can lead to abuses both through the practice of witchcraft on vulnerable persons and through witch-hunts against people believed to possess demonic powers. Twins and people with albinism are among those at risk from witches because their body parts are thought to have magical properties as medicine. According to a report produced for the United Nations High Commissioner for Refugees in 2011, thousands of people accused of witchcraft – mainly older women and children – are persecuted, tortured and murdered every year. Precise figures are understandably hard to come by, although a study by the Witchcraft and Human Rights Information Network, claimed to be the first systematic attempt to assess the scale of the problem worldwide, concluded that at least 865 people were murdered or harmed by witchcraft practices and accusations during 2013, based solely on reports in English-language media. The beliefs that lead to these atrocities are based in local traditions, but are often exacerbated by recent conflict as well as by the involvement of evangelical Christians from outside.

The British are not a people much given to trumpeting their virtues, but one thing we do like to tell ourselves is how tolerant we are. Tolerance is part of our national myth. In other countries, notably the United States, personal freedoms are more clearly protected by law, and so there is perhaps less need to bang on about tolerance. But tolerance can only be protected so far by law. Ultimately, it must be held as a good thing by the people.

In the early years of the twenty-first century, we are conflicted about this. Many quickly take offence when their beliefs or prejudices are challenged; we are told we must respect the views of minorities. The uneasy stand-off between offence and respect is a long way from true tolerance. It suggests in fact that we are basically intolerant, although we may be prepared temporarily to muzzle our intolerance. Count the things we tell ourselves we have zero tolerance for – drugs, terrorism, law-breaking, anti-social behaviour, bullying – and we quickly find ourselves confronting what is known as the tolerance paradox: how to tolerate those who are intolerant.

We deal with this difficulty largely by avoidance. Like most people, I try to arrange my life so that my tolerance of my fellow human being is not tested too forcefully. In that way I can then proclaim how tolerant I am. Thomas Browne undoubtedly pursued the same strategy in more trying circumstances. If I hear views that I regard as unacceptable, it is most likely to be through the media. My answering outrage at this can only be manufactured; it does not have the authenticity of spontaneous shock at a remark delivered face to face.

The tendency is to congratulate ourselves on how tolerant we are rather than to consider how much more tolerant we might be. In the seventeenth century, boiling alive and hand amputation were no longer the legal punishments for poisoning and publishing books hostile to the crown, for example. The practice of serfdom had recently lapsed. But it was still, as we have seen, more than respectable to believe in witches. We tolerate 'witches' now because we understand that they are merely people unlucky enough to find themselves at the margin of society, unfairly judged for living alone or exhibiting unusual appearance or behaviour. How do we now learn to tolerate, say, paedophiles? Pretending they do not exist or do not matter – the strategy of previous generations – will not do. But neither will the tabloids' option of calling them evil scum. We need to understand that paedophilia is not an evil, nor even an illness (with the implication of a medical cure), but a species of human behaviour, however hard that is to accept, and then to limit our sanctions against paedophiles to curtailing harm rather than exacting retribution that is fuelled by fears of our own subconscious.

We might be inclined to bask in self-righteousness at the progress we have made, but the greatest test of tolerance is to make the forward comparison, to look back at ourselves now from the future, and to discern the unquestioned justice that will seem by then cruel and inhuman. Even the greatest minds of Browne's age never imagined a day when slavery was abolished, when there was freedom of religion, when the vote might extend to women.

We might start with some basics. Is disability (mental as well as physical) fully accepted, when the disabled must be roughly 'assessed' for their eligibility to receive government benefits? Are the elderly treated with true equality by healthcare systems? Are the young treated fairly by the adults who fear them and envy their liberty? Of the four economic freedoms of the European Union – the free movement of capital, goods, services and people – it is not hard to see that it is the people who get the short straw (evident not least in the pernicious rhetoric of the moment which redefines people as workers, thereby reducing those who are not working to a subhuman level). Does a human have the right to deny another human liberty by imprisoning them? Does our love of meritocracy blind us to the inequality at its heart that leaves the stupid, lazy and feckless at a perpetual disadvantage?

Would it be going too far to predict a measure of animal equality? As I write, Steven Wise of the Nonhuman Rights Project has filed a habeas corpus suit on behalf of the captive chimpanzees of New York State, where he has discovered that the legal definition of 'personhood' is not explicitly limited to *Homo sapiens*. The notion of animal trials would have been nothing strange to Browne, when animals were occasionally brought to court for crimes of murder, injury and destroying crops. (These days, by comparison, when a dog mauls a child, it is usually put down with no such formality – is that progress?) In the very year in which Amy Denny and Rose Cullender were hanged at Bury, for example, a man called Potter was executed in New Haven, Connecticut, for 'damnable Bestialities', according to the redoubtable Cotton Mather, but not before he had been forced to see hang his guilty partners in the crime, 'a cow, two heifers, three sheep and two sows'.

7
Faith

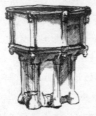

'the civility of my knee'

Religio Medici

IN ADDITION TO the cathedral and the castle known to Browne, Norwich now boasts a brick city hall with a copper-capped clock tower, a meagre emulation of the architectural masterpiece that is Stockholm City Hall. By means of these three landmarks, you can find your path through the tissue of lanes and alleys that run out from the Market Place, although your success at navigating in this way is liable to be hampered by more recent changes made for the benefit of road traffic.

Framing the city hall as you look across the square is the black knapped flint Guildhall on the right and the city's parish church of St Peter Mancroft on the left, built like the cathedral of imported stone, and with all the architectural bells and whistles the wool-swaddled fifteenth century could afford. It is a building 'more rich than aesthetically successful,' according to Nikolaus Pevsner. Facing the church today is the more disciplined modern brick Forum, which contains the regional offices of the BBC and Britain's most used public library. Civic pride would surely lead Browne to praise these buildings as he once did the cathedral, 'a handsome and well proportion'd fabrick, and one of the highest in England'. It is lower than Salisbury cathedral, he admits, but that building is only higher because its spire has been built on a taller tower above the crossing. Norwich's 'spire considered by itself seemes at least to equall that'.

Aside from these, Norwich has few grand civic edifices – no great post office, no imposing bank, no fearsome courthouse. The main theatre is inoffensively modern. The opera house? This is East Anglia, not Yorkshire. The one or two corporate headquarters are discreetly tucked away. Even the shopping centres are cleverly woven into much older urban fabric, one burrowing into Castle Mound, another reached by a path through a graveyard.

Today, it happens that the streets are crawling with Freemasons, beetle-like in their black suits, each carrying his mysterious flat case of regalia, on their way to some convocation. On the Soane bridge over the Wensum, I pass a hapless pair of Jehovah's Witnesses importuned by a doubter looking for an argument. The city seems quite other-century in this moment.

I have chosen to dally on this graveyard pathway by St Stephen's Church on my way to the Chapelfield shopping centre, where I have business at the Apple Store. I reckon it is a good place to observe the reaction of passers-by confronted by reminders of mortality. But it's not. They are oblivious, or if not, they are unfazed by the headstones, entirely focused on their mission of retail therapy.

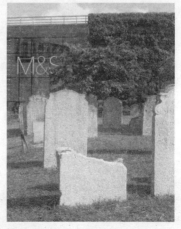

Unusually the church has all its doors flung wide. It is busy with excessively cheerful young men and women who purport to be running a cafe. It is a pilot project of an evangelical organization calling itself Norwich Youth for Christ. They plan to be there for a few days each week throughout the summer. It is a perfect pitch. They estimate that

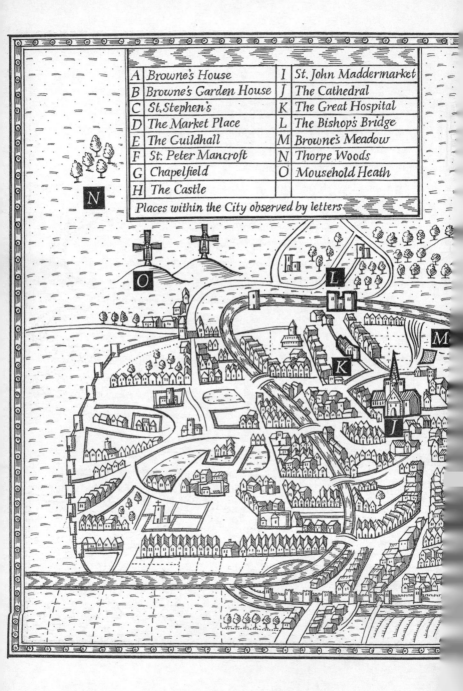

A	Browne's House	I	St. John Maddermarket
B	Browne's Garden House	J	The Cathedral
C	St. Stephen's	K	The Great Hospital
D	The Market Place	L	The Bishop's Bridge
E	The Guildhall	M	Browne's Meadow
F	St. Peter Mancroft	N	Thorpe Woods
G	Chapelfield	O	Mousehold Heath
H	The Castle		

Places within the City observed by letters.

NORWICH

50,000 people pass by in a week, 50,000 potential soldiers for Christ. They want me too.

'I'm pretty much an atheist,' I hear myself explaining, trying to inject the regretful tone that will tell them both that they are wasting their time and that I do not wish to be impolite. It sounds like an apology. Afterwards, I wonder why I did not simply say I am an atheist and leave it at that. I realize it is because it might seem confrontational, aggressive, dogmatic. Would an adjective have softened the blow? It would not have occurred to me to say, as some do, that I am a 'committed atheist'. I have experienced no process of committal. I just am an atheist, and that's all. It's part of me that doesn't take up much space. There is no ongoing dedication on my part. It's not that I am wavering; I *am* committed. It's just that I'm not committed in the way that Richard Dawkins is committed, in terms of devoting vast amounts of energy to an atheist project.

I don't believe in God or a god. Yet I am uncomfortable with declared atheism. Why is this? Am I in fact agnostic – that weasel word of English compromise for someone who isn't sure? Am I? No: I actually disbelieve.

Round here, I am not alone. The national census of England and Wales conducted in 2011 showed Norwich to be, as newspapers gleefully reported a few days before Christmas, the most godless city in the country. Norwich Youth *against* Christ, anybody? Just 44.9 per cent of people in the local authority area put Christian as their religion, while 42.5 per cent ticked the box for 'No religion'. The national averages were 59.3 per cent and 25.2 per cent respectively. Nationally, the number of people giving Christianity as their religion fell by more than 10 per cent from the previous census in 2001 (the first time it was thought interesting to include a question on religion). The numbers saying they have no religion rose by a similar percentage. Inevitably called upon for his comment, the Bishop of Norwich suggested that the census made it easier to say no than yes to the religion question ('No religion' was the first option on the checklist), and complained, oddly, I thought, for a faith leader, that there was no provision for people to position themselves where they felt they belonged on a spectrum of interest in religion.

I have other atheist credentials, too. Scientists and science writers are some of the most militant atheists around. From time to time, members of science academies are polled about their religious beliefs. According to one recent American study, about a third claim some form of belief in a higher power. A 1998 study published in *Nature*, cited by Richard Dawkins, found that the proportion of believers is dramatically less among more senior scientists. Among those elected to the National Academy of Sciences, only 7 per cent believed in a personal god.

Though he might wonder about God's bottom – 'we are ignorant of the backparts, or lower side of his Divinity' – Browne knows that scientific enquiry must have a stop. 'How shall the dead arise, is no question of my faith; to beleeve onely possibilities, is not faith, but meere Philosophy; many things are true in Divinity, which are neither inducible by reason, nor confirmable by sense.'

The popular perception that science and religion are at war is as old as modernity, but it was given its present character by the Oxford evolution debate in 1860, a few months after the publication of Darwin's *On the Origin of Species*. On this now famous occasion, Samuel Wilberforce, the Bishop of Oxford, took on 'Darwin's bulldog', Thomas Huxley. Was it from his grandfather or his grandmother that Huxley claimed his descent from an ape, the bishop wanted to know. Huxley struggled to be heard amid the hilarity and it seems that Wilberforce had the best of it on the night.

The debate is back in the spotlight more than a century later, prompted by who knows what – the advent of space travel, the ecological crisis, sectarian conflicts, a rise in Christian fundamentalism? This time it seems the boot is on the other foot, with religion finding no coherent answer to the trenchant arguments of scientific atheists such as Carl Sagan and Richard Dawkins. To follow their logic, it would seem that there should be neither religious scientists nor believers who value the principles of science.

In fact, the 'war' is greatly exaggerated. Scientists and religionists seldom cross paths, let alone swords. Many believers are also scientific rationalists and many scientists are also believers. But it will not rest there. For some scientists who are also atheists, other scientists who have a religious belief are something that needs to be explained. When these scientists investigate religion, they do so, naturally, in their usual scientific way, approaching religion as a social construct (although they seldom concede that science is also one). They may discover, through magnetic resonance imaging scans, for example, that there is nothing to be seen in a believing subject's brain that is any different from ordinary human emotion. Or they may argue that religious belief needs to be understood in terms of evolutionary biology. These endeavours might one day lay bare religious belief in terms of biology, and therefore ultimately in the materialist terms of chemistry and physics. But what would we really understand the better for having gone down this road?

You get more straightforward answers if you simply ask the scientists themselves. Some turn to religion because they believe science has shown the universe – through the numerical values of the fundamental constants of physics, the position of our planet, and so on – to be ideally suited for our existence. More interesting are those scientists, who often start out as religious sceptics, but who find that science offers no adequate explanation of phenomena such as beauty, truth and love. Theirs is not a choice for faith, against reason, but an attempt to reconcile the two. For influential figures such as the Hungarian chemist and philosopher Michael Polanyi or John Polkinghorne, a theoretical physicist later ordained as an Anglican priest, science and religion reveal different facets of the same reality. What we know is inevitably personal to us, they argue. This is the case even for scientific theories and mathematical axioms, since our conviction that they are true because they are seen to work is also personally apprehended. Scientific belief therefore finds itself on level terms with religious belief.

The Islamic fundamentalist attacks of 11 September 2001 helped to create a new audience for atheism. Books by Sam Harris, Daniel Dennett and Christopher Hitchens as well as Dawkins (they have been dubbed the 'four horsemen of the non-apocalypse') argued that religious faith could or should be brought to an end. Dawkins made himself the cheerleader of the 'new atheists' when he set up the Richard Dawkins Foundation for Reason and Science to hasten the day. His book *The God Delusion* makes the argument at length, but it is his frequent sulphurous outbursts on Twitter that better illustrate the furious tenor to which the spat (at this level it certainly cannot be called a debate) between religion and science has risen.

Sample Tweet: 'If one person claimed that a wafer was literally the body of a 1st century Jew, you'd certify him. That's what Catholics officially believe.' First of all, if a person claimed this, you wouldn't actually certify him (or her) for this harmless delusion under any reasonable mental health legislation; which means this is a gratuitous insult. Second, it's not quite what Catholics believe in any case: the bread and wine remain bread and wine (if one were rude enough to interpose a chemical analysis, say), but in the act of consecration their substance is changed into the substance of the body of Christ; according to the Catechism, it is a mode of His presence. Scientists may well have trouble with this, but semioticians will have less. Third, if it is what Catholics believe, then it is what they truly believe, not what they 'officially believe', a phrase that unreasonably projects Dawkins's own distrust into the minds of these believers.

Because of his combative language, and because his religiose scientism is so curiously like the fundamentalism he is attacking, Dawkins himself has become a target for abuse, although his supporters claim this is only because the believers can find no answer to his logic. Dawkins's bracing asperities are now routinely met in kind: 'Puffed up, self-regarding, vain, prickly and militant' was one columnist's string of adjectives for him.

My problem is that I agree more often with Richard Dawkins than with the Archbishop of Canterbury or the Pope, yet it is Dawkins who irritates me more. I am not looking for a middle ground – on the Bishop of Norwich's spectrum of interest in religion I am still at the not-interested end – but I wonder if a more civil accommodation can be reached between religion and science.

The signs are not good. Consider what happened when the geneticist Steve Jones published his recent book *The Serpent's Promise: The Bible Retold as Science*. Jones dares to look at the Bible as a kind of record of early attempts to understand the world, in other words as a work of science, in which Genesis is a story of the origin of the universe and Leviticus reflects sensible dietary precaution. For this, he was treated to some vituperative criticism from Christians unhappy at seeing stories they were used to regarding as allegory or metaphor treated as if they might actually have had a basis in physical fact. At the end of his trek through 'Dawkins's Canyon' – his name for the chasm between science and religion – Jones was forced to the odd conclusion that he in fact believes more of the Bible than many Christians do.

Browne's footprints also run through Dawkins's Canyon, for in *Religio Medici* and *Pseudodoxia Epidemica* he similarly considers possible natural origins of many biblical phenomena. Unlike Jones, Browne usually leans in the end towards the standard supernatural interpretation, even though he is fully aware of a plausible physical explanation. For example, he entertains the notion that the fire that consumes the altar of Elijah (1 Kings 18) might be a geological eruption of flammable naphtha or bitumen, which he has seen used in experiments. But he swiftly rejects the idea as the suggestion of the devil, and affirms the Bible story conclusion.

Thomas Browne's best-known statement of his faith is made at the very beginning of *Religio Medici*:

> For my Religion, though there be severall circumstances that might perswade the world that I have none at all, as the generall scandall of my profession, the naturall course of my studies, the indifferency of my behaviour, and discourse in matters of Religion, neither violently defending one, nor with that common ardour and contention opposing another; yet in despight hereof I dare, without usurpation, assume the honorable stile of a Christian.

It is a superb sentence first of all, with each phrase patiently shaped and placed in sequence in such a way as to postpone the end so that, when it comes, it has the requisite drama of confession. We are given the time to admire the way each part is carved, to feel how it weighs against the next part, before we draw back and gain the depth of perspective to see it assembled as a whole composition. Yet Browne's construction is still more artful than this. The sentence has not in fact been *assembled* in this way, for no part can now be removed without causing the whole thing to collapse. It has instead been organically hewn. Perhaps we experience something of the same disbelief before a wood carving by Grinling Gibbons when we realize that each exquisite detail has not been made separately and then added in, but rather its negative has been painstakingly chipped away to leave us with the final illusion of piled-up riches. It is in *Religio Medici*, according to Rose Macaulay, that Browne made 'in the most exquisite and splendid prose of the century, the best and most agreeable confession of the Anglican religion ever, before or since, published'.

In this affirmation, it is perhaps surprising that Browne considers it is not only his medicine – seen as suspect long before the seventeenth century began anatomizing the soul – but also his scientific hobby ('the naturall course of my studies') that leaves him open to charges of atheism. For the pursuit of scientific knowledge, to Browne, has the moral force almost of an article of faith.

Browne does not immediately say what form of Christianity he follows – a crucial matter for a young man widely travelled in Europe, and recently returned to an England where the king had asserted divine right and was fighting Catholic rebellion in Ireland and Presbyterian resistance in Scotland. But a few pages later he daringly comes out with this: 'I borrow not the rules of my Religion from *Rome* or *Geneva*, but the dictates of my own reason.' For this, *Religio Medici* soon found itself on the papal index.* In short, his faith was supple as it had to be, firmly

---

* Although he acknowledges that as an Anglican he is automatically a heretic excommunicated from the Church of Rome, Browne nevertheless writes that all people 'owe the duty of good language' to the Pope, and insists that he never

based in a conservative Anglicanism, yet adaptable to the requirements of the Commonwealth. It is impossible to doubt his basic loyalty to the Church of England when he deadpans that he has submitted all Churches to reasonable analysis and has found this is the one that comes out on top.

The first book of *Pseudodoxia Epidemica* itemizes the many sources of error that lead people to believe foolish things. The final cause Browne gives – after unreliable authors and credulous auditors – is the devil himself, who niggles at our mental weakness in numerous ways: 'he would make us believe, That there is no God, That there are many, That he himself is God, That he is less then angels or Men, That he is nothing at all'. Satan is not only the direct progenitor of error, but also the automatic supporter of those who promote errors of their own. Pseudoscience is the devil's work for Browne far more literally than it is for Dawkins or Simon Singh, today's scourge of homoeopaths and chiropractors. And God and science find themselves allies.

Elsewhere, Browne's Christian faith leads him towards a moral philosophy that would surely be acceptable to persons of any religion – or none. *Christian Morals*, a late work not published until long after Browne's death, might be expected to be a summation of his religion. And in a way it is, as the Christian message quickly gives way to a charac- teristic humanism, mingled with advice on how to go about things if, as it happens, you are a person a bit like Browne. The first few of seventy- nine numbered paragraphs begin with admonishments against the seven deadly sins – 'Let Age not Envy draw wrinkles on thy cheeks' for example. But soon, Browne is blandly recommending moderation in all things and telling us how to handle wealth and flattery. Much of it

---

'returned to his the name of Antichrist, Man of sin, or whore of Babylon', as he presumably had heard others do in England. It cannot have helped that he put these epithets in print in *Religio Medici*, however, even in self-exculpation. On the *Index of Prohibited Books*, Browne found himself in the excellent company of Rabelais, Galileo, Bacon, Hobbes and Spinoza.

is completely secular advice on how to live that anybody might wish to follow: be your own master, be generous, try to see the good in everybody, don't listen to gossip, be grateful for small mercies. It is all highly uncontroversial, an anodyne bookend to the protean *Religio Medici*. For a modern equivalent, I recommend the philosophical works of Alain de Botton and his School of Life.

A few of the aphorisms contained in *Christian Morals* have a startling modern air: one might now be paraphrased as 'respect difference'; another as 'be yourself'. But of course Browne says it all uncommonly well. He offers the tritest of marriage advice – don't go to bed angry – as follows: 'Let not the Sun in Capricorn go down upon thy wrath, but write thy wrongs in Ashes. Draw the Curtain of night upon injuries, shut them up in the Tower of Oblivion and let them be as though they had not been.' He counsels us not to blame the stars; to study history, not predictions; and to act our age. One especially fine paragraph exhorts us not to waste time:

> Since thou hast an Alarum in thy Breast, which tells thee thou hast a Living Spirit in thee above two thousand times in an hour; dull not away thy Days in sloathful supinity & the tediousness of doing nothing. To strenuous Minds there is an inquietude in overquietness, and no laboriousness in labour; and to tread a mile after the slow pace of a Snail, or the heavy measures of the Lazy of Brazilia [the sloth], were a most tiring Pennance, and worse than a Race of some furlongs at the Olympicks.

And in the midst of all, he throws in some invaluable advice to scholars and writers: avoid academicism; don't be too harsh on other people's mistakes; risk being wrong for the sake of bringing new knowledge to the world; don't sweat the small stuff, or rather: 'if the substantial subject be well forged out, we need not examine the sparks, which irregularly fly from it'.

With his humanistic ethics and his dangerous medicine and science, would Browne be an atheist today? He offers the occasional hint that it is not inconceivable. He sometimes writes of Christians with a critical distance, as if he is not one himself. He writes about those 'such as hope to rise again', implying perhaps that he does not expect a Christian resurrection for himself. He even confesses in *Urne-Buriall* to a sneaking admiration for men 'such as consider none hereafter'; for these – whether believers in other religions, pre-Christians or non-believers – 'it must be more than death to dye, which makes us amazed at those audacities, that durst be nothing, and return into their *Chaos* again'.

But when he tackles the matter directly, he says there can be no such thing as atheism, or at least there can be no 'positive atheists'. For some philosophers who might be thought atheists, Browne goes to some lengths to find a reason why they were not. Epicurus was no atheist when he denied there was a beneficent god, for example; it is simply that the God of Christians was 'too sublime' to make himself known to him. The Stoics were also subject, without their knowing it, to God's will, and so are no atheists either. Besides, it is the devil, as we have seen, who plants atheistic thoughts.

It is hard now to recreate a sense of the almost complete impossibility of not being a religious believer in seventeenth-century England. But as I enter the Apple Store, symmetrically laid out with its central entrance door and an attractively illuminated high table at the far end, a parallel comes to mind. Digital technology seems to fill a large part of the mental space we reserve for faith. (Art, which is often put up as a candidate, is the opium only of a minority.) We depend on technology for the smooth running of our daily lives, if not for our salvation. We make obeisance to it, we feel obliged to buy into the whole package, rather than selecting and rejecting individual technologies. There is the familiar choice between minutely differentiated sects (Apple or Microsoft), but all must share the same basic creed. Upgrades are like revisions of dogma in which we have no say, but which we are bound to go along with anyway. To reject the technological is to declare oneself a heretic, a position as inconceivable now as declaring oneself an atheist in the 1600s.

To be an atheist now seems almost too easy. I have nothing against church architecture or decent sacred music. The aesthetic is fine. My problem with the Christian faith comes when my ear snags on something the preacher has just said, and I make the mistake of thinking about what it might actually mean. On the radio, I take exception to the simpering neediness of English vicars ('O Lord, make speed to save us' – Yes, Lord, look sharp). 'Thought for the Day' on the radio morning news is usually a good moment to run a bit more hot water into the bath.

Knowing how I feel, my wife gave me Dawkins's *The God Delusion* for Christmas when it came out in 2006, but it soon found its way to the bedside table where it languishes still (like a hotel-room Gideon's Bible?). A marker indicates that I got as far as page seventy-eight. I have not felt the urge to attend the Festival of Nine Lessons and Carols for Godless People, a Christmas-time theatrical event hosted by the comedian Robin Ince, and organized by *New Humanist* magazine. Nor the Sunday Assembly, 'a godless congregation that celebrates life', a strange initiative apparently desperate to keep all the non-liturgical bits of church services – the getting together, enjoying a singalong, hearing some words to make you think, everything, in fact, except actual belief in a god.

The Sunday Assembly's slogan is warm and vague: 'live better, help often, wonder more'. Of course, it sounds a bit religious. But the sentiments are secular, too. Who does not want to live better? And why should the religious have the monopoly when it comes to being charitable (a monopoly some believers are keen to retain, to judge by recent reports of atheists being barred from helping in food banks)? What about 'wonder more'? What is wonder? Is it admiration of the intricacy and complexity of nature, and the potential for it to be understood; or is it throwing in the towel, admitting there are things that cannot be understood at which we can only wonder? What bothers me most, though, is the air of superiority hanging about the slogan. I can imagine that people who self-consciously go around living better, helping often and wondering more might be just as self-righteous as the worst sort of Christian moralist.

These efforts by science to eclipse religion are one thing. Elsewhere, there are initiatives to seek a rapprochement between the two. Seeing a market opportunity if not an intellectual one, many universities have set up centres for the joint study of science and religion. And in 2012, the discovery of the Higgs boson – the supposed 'God particle' – prompted the European nuclear research centre, CERN, to organize a high-level conference of theologians, physicists and philosophers.

With all this ferment, I begin to wonder if the way in which Browne chooses intellectually to accommodate his faith alongside his scientific reason, far from being a cop-out, isn't in fact a rather subtle and profound settlement that offers some resolution in a futile war. Science and faith, each has its moment and each has its method. His philosophical doubts he reasons out, Browne tells us in *Religio Medici*; his religious doubts, though, he conquers 'not in a martiall posture, but on my knees'.

He has simply put science in one place to be dealt with in one way, and religion in another place to be dealt with in another way. His implacable illogic maddens me, and yet somehow I admire him for it, too. Dawkins and his allies know that faith is absurd to reason and hit a brick wall. Browne knows that faith is absurd to reason and accepts the fact. Indeed, he runs with it. What does he gain? He immediately sees that the world, and the texts that describe it, are more interesting, rich, confusing and ambiguous because they contain more than literal truth. Dawkins is like Francis Bacon, who wanted a word to be assigned safely to each material thing, but Browne knows that words and the world are not true – not entirely. His religion is not a rational way to understand the world but it is a poetic, mythic and metaphoric one. It bestows on him a tolerance when confronted by those less enlightened than himself, not ire and frustration. It predisposes him to seriousness before mystery, not flippancy.

I am passing his statue again. Would it be too much for him to climb down from his plinth? Probably it is. But here he comes,

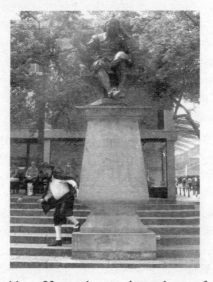

Commendatore-like…He gently puts down the pot fragment he has been cupping in his right hand, and steps nimbly off his plinth by the belt man's stall on Hay Hill.

TB: Phew. You would not believe the piaculous things I have seen from up there. The vulgar people of Norwich do not much change. You are writing about me, I understand.

HAW: Yes. Even in Norwich, people know little about you. I did a vox pop – a survey of people right here. Most had no idea who you were, I'm afraid to say. A few thought you were Shakespeare.

TB: I do not know whether to be flattered or distressed. Even this fine statue is too much for me. Ah, it is good to be on the vulgar plane once more. The aerial view can exhaust one.

HAW: I feel you have lessons for our century, which is the twenty-first, by the way.

TB: So, is this some kind of bromance?

HAW: I see you have not lost your interest in novel words.

TB: I have had much time to listen.

HAW: We could go to Pret a Manger…

TB: Pret a…? I am not ready to manger. My house! It stood on this spot, I think. The place at least has changed in futurity, and much beyond our imaginary estimations. No, let us make a tollutation about my old city as we talk.

HAW: There will be much you will still recognize. I particularly wanted to speak to you about religion and science. We seem to have got ourselves into a spot of difficulty with the two.

TB: I sense, though, that this is not a matter of great personal concern for you. You are a mere observer of stormy weather, I think. As for yourself, you were born in England a Christian?

HAW: I was not born with any religion, of course. But, er, yes, I was christened, although I had no say in it. I have no religion. I was married in church too, before you ask. Some things in life it is important to do in the exact way that others have done them before. Ritual must be shared to be meaningful, and it seems churches have the monopoly, or at least the track record, of providing this ritual.

TB: You are an atheist then. There are those who thought me so.

HAW: I am not sure my unbelief is active enough to merit an -ism. It takes up little of my thought. But, yes.

TB: Am I here to explain why I am no atheist, and would be not so even in your heathen day, or to explain to you why you are an atheist? Perhaps we should begin by finding where we agree. We agree that the pursuit of knowledge of the world through science is a virtue. I believe it leads people out of Error that came after the Fall. I'm not sure why you're so keen. For what your age deludes itself is progress? No? For curiosity's sake, then. We can agree that much remains unknown, and this is something exciting. When did you begin to doubt, or did you never believe?

HAW: No event that I can recall. Just a gradual growing disdain for the flabbiness of the Church of England. Perhaps Northern Ireland and the Middle East were a factor as I was growing up. In the C. of E., it seems it doesn't really matter if you believe or not. That should help me, but I find it puzzling. Out of architectural curiosity, I once visited a big London mosque, and was set upon – that seems almost the right phrase – by enthusiastic young men, who had spotted me as an anomaly and a potential recruit. They were still more astonished when my atheism came to light. Perhaps some of them were genuinely appalled. Anyway, I extricated myself with difficulty. That never happens in an English cathedral.

TB: I wonder if you became more an atheist as you became more a scientist. As I can relate, the one need not proceed with the other in correlation.

HAW: I suppose so. But I do understand that science and religion meet different needs and seek to answer different questions. I see that belief is a larger field than knowledge, and what lies beyond the bounds of knowledge is not necessarily either negligible or uninteresting.

TB: But others in your time do not, I see. Ah, here is the cathedral. It is looking better than in my rebellious times when the burial places of so many noble persons were desecrated. The tombs are the true life of the place. When do you think you come closest to religious feeling?

HAW: I am not overwhelmed by the urge to believe when I walk into a cathedral, although I do admire the strength of the vision that put it there. Hearing *The Messiah* might bring me closer to what I suppose you are talking about.

TB: Hearing the Messiah! Methinks it would.

HAW: *The Messiah* is an oratorio by a composer called Handel, born a couple of years after you, uh, died. Yes, sublime music comes close. I read a moving account of a man suddenly reinforced in his belief by hearing Mozart's *Clarinet Concerto* in a cafe. I suspect, though, that the emotions of someone undergoing what they feel is a religious experience are just the same as those felt by an unbelieving listener like me.

TB: My difficulty is this. We both accept there is mystery. You believe that all mystery will potentially yield itself unto science; I do not.

I believe there are things unknown that by their very unknown-ness may not stand to be known in the ways of our science. This makes atheism the greatest falsity. To affirm there is no God is the highest lie in nature. Besides, there never was any absolute atheist who could prove there is no God.

HAW: I see. I hesitate to say this. Perhaps you should move on. You have been dogmatically wrong before. Need I mention the witch trial? It's actually all right to be an atheist now. In fact, Norwich is the most godless place in the country. Even the present Pope has said that atheists are 'acceptable' and may be redeemed if they do good. At any rate, my issue is not with atheism per se, but with those who have been labelled New Atheists.

TB: They sound like the New Model Army.

HAW: I dislike the tone, and sometimes the content, of the argument that has arisen between them and the religious community. It has become unpleasantly **ferocious**.

TB: Ha! I see some words of my coinage are still on common tongues.

HAW: Ferocious? Yes. In this rush to the extremes, both atheists and believers must strenuously assert their positions. The faith must be observed by the book. Or the science must be the whole answer. There is no middle ground.

TB: I fear you are exaggerating. Even in my time of civil war and reli-gious strife there were many who were but the passivest Christians. My own belief, as you know, is far from literal, and based on the law of mine own reason as well as upon Grace. There is far greater freedom in your time. Or do these New Atheists wish to

---

※-※-※-※-※-※-※-※-※-※ ※ ※ ※-※-※-※-※-※-※-※-※-※

ferocious (PE, 1646): Browne calls the lion 'a fierce and ferocious animal', immediately raising the question of what 'ferocious' means that is not already covered by 'fierce'. Both words stem from the Latin *ferus*, meaning wild, but 'ferocious' comes to us via the Latin derivative of *ferus*, *ferox*, which means wild-looking. The lion is undoubtedly both wild and wild-looking, fierce and ferocious. Other creatures might be fierce, but not ferocious, or ferocious, but not fierce.

enforce atheism among the people? Do you? Would you wish to
see religious belief wither from the earth? Or, without that evasive
conditionality, and to come to the point, do you wish to see it go?

HAW: You mean: do I wish to see what Dawkins calls the 'virus of
religion' eradicated? I suppose I am bound to say yes. But with
numerous caveats. I would safeguard the cultural goods religion
has conferred: the art and architecture, the music, even the Bible
and the other sacred books that cause such trouble. I would not
destroy these things as your age often did, and as happens still
in some countries today. And I have no wish to force the pace
– that would be too much like religious zealotry itself. Nor am
I so naive as to fall for the idea that any of this would end the
conflicts and wars that we presently characterize as religious; I am
sure many of them would rise again dressed in different ideologies. Nor do I believe in a wholly atheist society any more than a
wholly Christian or Jewish or Muslim one. Atheism is a matter
for individuals. But if fewer in each generation feel the need to
believe, as seems to be happening here and there – especially here,
as I say – then I welcome it. It would certainly be good to see the
back of the unaccountable patriarchies that control the ways in
which people are allowed to engage with their gods.

TB: What would you actually do?

HAW: I would argue rationally when challenged. But it is not for me to
make converts.

TB: I suppose atheism cannot be enforced as faith cannot be enforced.
Certainly, I do not think it requisite to attempt it. It is no reasonable proceeding to compel a religion, or to think to enforce our
own belief upon another, if, without the concurrence of God's
spirit, they lack their own evidence of the things that are imposed.
So is it also in matters of common belief, where we cannot indubitably assent either, without the cooperation of our sense or
reason, which persuade us. For as the habit of faith in divinity
is an argument of things unseen, and a stable assent unto things

inevident, upon authority of the Divine Revealer, so the belief of man which depends upon human testimony is but a staggering assent unto the affirmative, not without some fear of the negative. And as there is required the word of God, or infused inclination unto it, so must the actual sensation of our senses, or at least the non opposition of our reasons, procure our assent and acquiescence in the other…

HAW: Sorry, you lost me there for a moment. So what you're saying is, without a leap of faith it's even harder to persuade people. The rationalists who want us to run our lives on evidence-based reasoning certainly have an uphill struggle in front of them. Or a staggering ascent. Ha, ha!

TB: I sometimes find my rebellious reason in league with Satan. But I find it helps when I assert my faith to recall what Tertullian said: *Certum est quia impossibile*. Oh, you do not speak Latin? 'It is certain because it is impossible.'

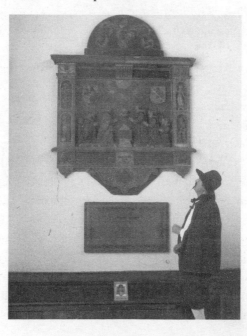

HAW: Ah yes, I have to say I have some trouble with this. You know Dawkins found this passage of yours, where you go on to say you seek out impossibilities as things to strengthen your faith. He calls it 'the "mystery is a virtue" infection'. 'That way madness lies,' he says. But in your case, you'll be glad to hear, Dawkins reckons 'something more interesting is going on here than just plain insanity or surrealist nonsense'. In the end, though, you only add to his outrage. You're worse than mad, you're pernicious for the way you imply that faith is some kind of game of one-upmanship in believing ever-greater impossibilities.

TB: I can only plead guilty. I do like to lose myself in a mystery and pursue my reason to an O altitudo! However, do not exclude the possibility that my hunger for greater and more impenetrable mysteries arises not only because they may be insoluble, but also because they may be soluble, and I will enjoy the unravelling of them. I am interested in both deliveries. Is this not the behaviour also of a philosophical mind?

HAW: You write that you are glad you never saw a miracle. That surprises me.

TB: It is true I believe in miracles. But I have no wish to see one. I am not entirely sure why. If I am honest, I fear it is because, if I were to witness one, I should not be able to forbear from making it into a philosophical exploration and … it might prove no miracle.

HAW: Of course Dawkins would demand to see the miracle to see if it conforms as a repeatable experiment.

TB: I am content to understand a mystery without a rigid definition. Many a Christian believes he has seen a miracle, too, and he finds this is a support to his faith. But occurrences can have meaning even if they do not demonstrably happen. It is an easy belief to credit what our eye hath examined, but harder that which lies beyond sense. Harder, but perhaps more worth the while.

HAW: Like the Big Bang and quantum phenomena perhaps? The American physicist Warren Weaver once said that science is 'based largely on faith in the reasonableness, order and beauty of the universe of which man is part'.

TB: I do not know about these things you name. But I can agree with that. I believe further that the humility of science may open the way to faith. Since I was of the understanding to think we knew nothing, I have found my reason hath been more pliable to the will of faith.

HAW: I can't go along with that. But I do see how an element of faith may be involved in ordinary matters of science. How do I know my readiness to connect this winter's storms with global climate change is not simply the equivalent of your century's explanation of storms as divine retribution? The same urge to draw a dire moral lesson is there. I know a little of the science that underpins the link. But I still have to have faith that the science is sound, and faith that I could, if called upon, find the right data to prove it. This isn't a religious faith, because the evidence is not actually absent, it is only inconveniently distant. But Weaver was referring to something deeper, I think. Science operates on the principle that the simple explanation is to be preferred to the complex, that simple mechanisms are the most tenacious, that fundamentally simple relationships govern the most complicated natural phenomena. Why must there be an explanation? Why do we feel it must be a simple one? This is the drive behind scientific reductionism as well as religious faith. Perhaps it all comes down to mathematics.

TB: Now this is a question meriting of a deuteroscopy. I am not equipped to offer mathematical truths, but I do find number everywhere mysteriously in nature. Here, let me pluck this houseleek from the wall. I can show you the quincunxial ordination of the thing. Of course, I ran off in all directions in my pursuit of quincunxes everywhere. Imagination is apt to rove, and conjecture keeps no bounds. *The Garden of Cyrus* was meant not only as a work of science. But your 'reasonableness, order and beauty' are all here in vegetable creation, which was the first ornamental scene in nature. Who made them ornament and not chaos? And with what spectator in mind? We find strict rules in the springing of seeds, and good economy in how little is required unto effectual generation. There is nothing useless in nature, as Montaigne tells us. Nature is the art of God, but it is also a productive engine. We divine, too, that there must be some undiscerned principle that balances the production of variety in things.

HAW: We admire nature with a god or without. But if it is art, it is an art that is confrontational and tough. It forces us to think of cruelty and waste as well as beauty and simplicity. The principles that govern variety that you mention will come with a naturalist called Charles Darwin some 200 years after your time. His theory of natural selection will set all this out.

TB: But God is needed as a cause of all.

HAW: No, only millions of years of trial and error to refine each surviving species. Each generation passes on the minutest improvements to the next.

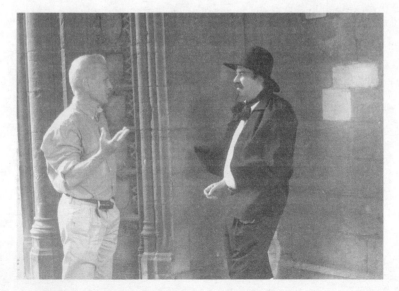

TB: Aha. Common men wonder why among millions no two look alike, while I had wondered that there should be any alike at all, since so many words can be made from twenty-six letters. Now I will properly understand the reason.

HAW: We'll stop off at the Book Hive and get you *On the Origin of Species*. You will enjoy it, but be appalled at the implications, as Darwin was himself.

TB: And then at last, when homeward I shall drive / Rich with the spoils of nature from th'Book Hive.

HAW: What?

TB: Oh. Nothing…

HAW: Perhaps they'll have some of Dawkins's books too.

TB: Dawkins, always Dawkins. Who is this saltimbanco?

HAW: A zoologist once, or zoographer as you had it. An enquirer after order in nature like you. But he has made himself into an atheist crusader with a book called *The God Delusion*.

TB: *The God Delusion?* Of course God is a kind of delusion. Even in my age, no man of learning believes there is a man with a white beard in the heavens. But it is a helpful image for vulgar heads to have, who do not understand a metaphor. I wonder, does Dawkins? He should take care lest he run into extremities from whence there is no regression. In the vicious ways of the world it mercifully falleth out that we become not extempore wicked, but it taketh some time and pains to undo our selves. But I must not quarrel with an adversary not yet understood else I overlook the mercies bound up in him.

HAW: Because of fundamentalist religion on the one hand and militant atheism on the other, we are being driven into corners where belief – in God, or in science – must be literal and unshakable.

TB: You might think that it was like this in my disturbed time too, but it was not always. Belief can be soft and flexible. I have experienced a few Christianities, and I have mixed mine own by commolition of their versions to satisfy mine own reason. Though the world be histrionical, and most men live ironically, you can be what you singly are, and personate only yourself.

HAW: That's good to know. Science and religious belief are both constrained by the senses, are they not? Is looking – scientific observation – not enough? Alternatively, why even bother to look if all will be revealed? You looked at everything. Why?

TB: I did look at many things, and wished to look at more. Surely, though, we cannot doubt there is something beyond what we can see. It is the purest conceit to think that the world reaches no further than the limits of our own senses, though many things conspire to make us think it does not. This noisome traffic, these shifting images, all these curious fellows and their mistresses, these cornucopious shops do greatly numb mine own apprehension in this very moment. Earthly things.

HAW: Do you believe in scientific progress?

TB: I am a tireless slave unto curiosity, and always ready to attend with patience the uncertainty of things, and what lieth yet unexerted in the chaos of futurity. Our ignorance of things to come makes the world new unto us by unexpected emergences, and the novelizing spirit of man lives by variety and the new faces of things. But to the notion that we might improve upon the world, I discover my brain anatomized in two halves, the one believing that it is my medical duty, the other knowing that the world will be brought to its end. For me, the purpose of what you call science is, as I said, to correct Error and to return mankind to our condition before the Fall. Is that not a progressive idea?

HAW: Um, not really, no. You expected the world to end quite soon, didn't you?

TB: I suppose I must confess I am surprised to find the end has not come yet. Which year is this? Twenty-what? Did not even the millennium produce some expectation of the resurrection of the dead?

HAW: A little. Yet here we are 330 years later. The prelapsarian ideal –

TB: My kind of word! I've not heard that one before.

HAW: The prelapsarian ideal is a bit out of fashion. What about the material betterment of humankind's condition in this life?

TB: Ah, well, 'tis better to think that times past have been better than times present, than that times were always bad. There is nothing more acceptable unto the ingenious world than the noble eluctation of truth wherein, against the tenacity of prejudice, my century did bravely begin to prevail. So many centuries were lost in sealing up the book of knowledge. Yet now what libraries of new volumes your and after times will behold.

HAW: What is this knowledge for? It is a chief article of faith – yes, I know, faith – of contemporary science that progress is in a forward direction.

TB: Yet is not the idea that man bears within him the fall of Adam a useful corrective to this human conceit?

HAW: I think it is not a helpful aspect of Christianity to be constantly told we are sinners. But do I believe that we are becoming less

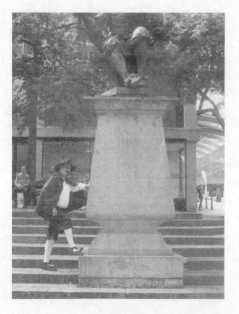

evil, as Steven Pinker insists in his book *The Better Angels of Our Nature*? Perhaps. But if so, not fast enough.

TB: Is this moral progress not attributable to the beneficence of the Christian religion?

HAW: Who knows? There is plenty to suggest that our supposed advance – moral and technological – is not always forward. I'm sorry, I'm a mass of contradictions on this…

TB: It is acceptable to be so. At least, I hope so, for I am too. Ah, here we are again. I wonder if you could give me a leg-up.

8
Melancholy

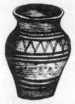

'sometimes not without morosity'

Religio Medici

Barrows and quoits and cairns are prominent on hilltops across counties in the west of the British Isles. But these ancient burial markers are absent from East Anglia. It is not because the country was not settled. It is because of the geology: there is not the stone to put up extravagant markers; there is soft chalk and lumpen flint suitable for no permanent memorial, and the light soil invites simpler inhumation.

It was not until the twentieth century that this earth began to reveal great treasures of its own. The Anglo-Saxon ship burial at Sutton Hoo – perhaps the resting place of the seventh-century East Anglian King Raedwald – was revealed on the eve of the Second World War. Then, in 1942, a farmer ploughing his field uncovered the Mildenhall hoard of Roman silver. These Suffolk finds were followed in 1979 by the excavation of Spong Hill at North Elmham in Norfolk, the largest Anglo-Saxon burial site known.

It is easy, then, to see why Thomas Browne might have been so excited by the discovery of some ancient burial remains in his own county. He rides across country to take a look, in spite of more pressing duties, and is immediately inspired to write what many consider to be his greatest

work of literature, *Urne-Buriall*, over the weeks that follow. In the dedicatory letter at the head of the work, he protests uninterest, but it is plain
he cannot resist the lure of ancient objects brought out into the light,
inviting his gaze and demanding description:

> We are coldly drawn unto discourses of Antiquities, who have scarce
> time before us to comprehend new things, or make out learned
> Novelties. But seeing they arose as they lay, almost in silence among
> us, at least in short account suddenly passed over; we were very
> unwilling they should die again, and be buried twice among us.

The precise location where forty or fifty urns were found is no longer
known. Nor is it known what has become of their contents, 'skulls, ribs,
jawes, thigh-bones, and teeth, with fresh impressions of their combustion', together with fragments of boxes, metal tools, combs and jewels.
The best description of the site is Browne's own, and he merely says that
they were found 'in a field of old Walsingham'. This is the small village
of Great Walsingham long
since eclipsed by the ironically larger pilgrimage
site of Little Walsingham,
which has a shrine to the
Virgin Mary dating from
the eleventh century. It is
a vast parish, and although
Browne says the soil was
dry and sandy and the depth of burial not greater than a yard, it is
impossible to know where to begin to look for the site.

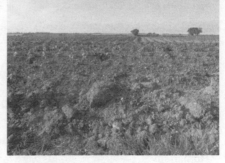

He breaks off from writing *The Garden of Cyrus*, his exploration of
nature rampant. The turn from life to death is nothing new to him,
of course. As a father and as a physician, he has seen it often enough.
And as a writer, he has hardly avoided the subject, musing on what
happens to the body and the soul in *Religio Medici*, and speculating in

Pseudodoxia Epidemica on the ages to which animals live, on unusual deaths of famous men, and on the sweet sound of the swan song.

But here it is different. Before, he was inquisitive, dispassionate and brisk. Death was chiefly a matter of biological fact. Gazing down at the body on the dissection bench, 'marshalling all the horrours, and contemplating the extremities thereof, I finde not any thing therein able to daunt the courage of a man, much lesse a well resolved Christian', he writes as a young man in *Religio Medici*. Now, at the age of fifty-two, death becomes his muse. In *Urne-Buriall*, Browne embraces the paradoxes of human presence and loss, and the futility of our struggle to persist beyond our years, as those who were immemorial suddenly demand to be remembered: 'Time which antiquates Antiquities, and hath an art to make dust of all things, hath yet spared these *minor* Monuments. In vain we hope to be known by open and visible conservatories, which to be unknown was the means of their continuation and obscurity their protection…'

His topic is in tune with the times. Melancholia was the cultural fashion. 'In the sixteenth and seventeenth centuries,' according to the

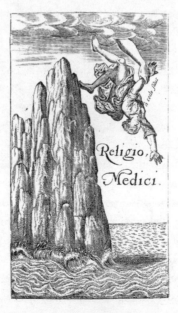

sociologist Bryan Turner, 'England was renowned for the melancholic disposition of its inhabitants; a special term was coined – "the English malady" to describe the prevalence of this national sickness.' Various reasons have been proposed for this, from the slaughter of the Civil War to the religious and political uncertainties that they stirred. But does fashion need a reason? What is clear is that the genre was well established by the time Browne came on the scene, set in train by the tearful songs of the lutenist John Dowland, by Shakespeare's *Hamlet*, and by Robert Burton's colossal book *The Anatomy of Melancholy*, published in 1621. These were no outpourings of incoherent grief but the subtlest contemplations of life and death brought off with exquisite poise.

Urne-Buriall is certainly a prime example of the type. Burial urns are an amply maudlin subject. Their gaping volumes seem to speak what we cannot about the forgetting act of burial. However, the stimulus for the essay is not burial but an accidental disinterment, an unearthing, and it has in it also the promise of discovery. Unlike these other melancholic works, this has real evidence to put forward, authentic artefacts that Browne has seen, charred bones and the nameless vessels themselves that are emblematic of the emptied bodily vessel of life, but that also cry out for their rightful place to be known in science and history.

These opportune finds are another subject for Browne's insatiable curiosity, like a plant or an animal that has been brought to him, allowing him to display his learning in all its breadth and depth. The essay is prized for its baroque prose, but it is also a disciplined report of a scientific investigation.

He begins with a multicultural survey of funerary customs, looking in particular at the preference for burial or cremation, and keeping a sharp eye out for ironies – of the latter, he notes that Christians once 'abhorred this way of obsequies', but nevertheless would readily offer up victims to be burnt alive when the Spanish Inquisition was still at work. In the second chapter, Browne sets his scene at Walsingham, giving an outline description of the artefacts found there, although the urns themselves are mostly without inscriptions or other identifying features.

The shortage of conclusive evidence for the provenance of these remains leaves Browne free to do what he does best and to consider all possibilities. Enriching his narrative with references to accounts of some grand interments of Romans and Danes, he eventually narrows down a date for these urns to the Saxon period between these two.

The third chapter offers a fuller description of the urns, their design, their parts, and their charred human contents. Browne even tastes the metal fragments, and observes how, suddenly exposed to the air, they begin to corrode. He tells us how small is the quantity of ash that a human body produces, and speculates on the heat of combustion of human flesh: 'the *Saracens* burnt in large heaps, by the King of *Castile*, shewed how little Fuell sufficeth'. Once again, the pertinent details of these urns are all but lost amid stories of more famous burials, of Plato, Nero and Domitian, and of Childeric, king of the Franks. Browne perhaps hopes to aggrandize these Norfolk remains, but he risks reburying them with words.

In the final chapters, Browne allows his thoughts to wander freely. He lights upon another Christian irony in the concern for ritual around the body at death when it is the soul that really matters. He weighs the Epicurean position that there is no afterlife against the Christian promise of resurrection as fairly as he can. 'A Dialogue between two Infants in the womb concerning the state of this world, might handsomely illustrate our ignorance of the next', he writes. He ends on the vain paradox of our hoping to be remembered after death when everything essential about us has disappeared. Drawing towards his conclusion, Browne writes: 'man is a Noble Animal, splendid in ashes, and pompous in the grave'. It is perhaps his most quoted aphorism.* What do these adjectives really mean? It is a comment on our vanity, of course, but also the perceptive remark of a natural philosopher who

---

* The circulation of quotations from Browne has benefited from the advent of Twitter, where every day a few dozen of his shorter aphorisms are re-broadcast. The sentence that follows the one I have quoted, 'Life is a pure flame, and we live by an invisible sun within us', is also popular.

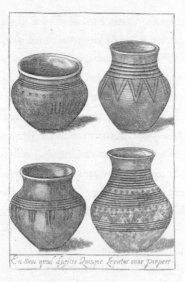

En Sum quod digitis Quinque Levatur onus propert

has observed that among all the animals we are the only creatures that exhibit the urge to self-commemorate.

Today, in the absence of the objects to which it refers, *Urne-Buriall* stands as a work of pure literature more than a scientific account. The spirit of enquiry that always guided Browne is more evident in his account of a similar find which is given with less thought for posterity.

By his own admission, he had not expected to return to the topic of funerary urns when, in 1667, a decade after the unearthing of the

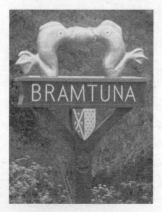

Walsingham urns, someone tells him of a new discovery on land close to the Pastons' seat at Oxnead Hall. He can hardly get there fast enough. In his short report, he describes the site with the infuriatingly vague precision of a pirate telling where buried treasure lies. These new urns lie in 'a large arable feild lying between Buxton and Brampton, but belonging unto Brampton and not much more then a furlong from Oxned park'.

He explains that they were found by workmen digging ditches during enclosure, the systematic taking of historical common land into private ownership that began in England in Tudor times and gathered pace during the Civil War.

Browne arrives while the diggers are still at work. Their discoveries have created quite a stir. Local people have joined them to scrabble through the soil for themselves to see what they can find. The workmen have broken the urns as they come across them in the earth, though, and finding nothing of interest within them, only ashes, have scattered the fragments. However, Browne notices two urns apparently still complete protruding from the sides of the ditch. He instructs the men to proceed with care to try to extract them whole, but these urns break too as they are released from the grip of the soil.

He takes them to be Roman or Romano-British. It is the first time they have breathed the air for more than a thousand years. These are objects from classical civilization reborn, actual objects, tangible comple-ments to Browne's prized classical texts. But do they speak? What can they tell us?

The urns vary in size, shape and colour. Browne reasons that the large ones may be family urns. Some have lids, others do not. Some are found upright, others with their necks pointing down. A few bear inscriptions, but most do not. The words cannot be made out. Are they the names of the interred, or those of the maker? Some genitive endings suggest the latter.

Other items are more revealing. People bring him Roman coins they have found. He is suddenly everybody's favourite expert on the *Antiques Roadshow*, as he explains to excited peasants the scarcely credible dates of the items they proffer and tells them stories of the figures they depict. The coins show Roman dignitaries from the second and the third centu-ries, indicating long occupation of the site.

Others digging nearby find something much larger: a square slab made of a brick-like material, pierced with holes. A couple of pots rest mouth down on two of these holes. Reaching through this perforated layer they find another similar layer below, and then three more below that, with a few more pots shelved here and there. Browne wonders if this is like some sites he has read about where holes are left for the insertion of the ashes of later generations. Any human remains, though, appear to have been thoroughly burnt, and all Browne can find are some pieces that he believes may be fragments of teeth. The rest is ash or formless black lumps. He sniffs and cannot forget the aroma.

After Walsingham, Browne is convinced that this, too, is a site of funerary ceremony, and launches once again into gloomy literary flight. He refutes those who think that, because many burial urns have been found in the past, there cannot be many more to be discovered. For Browne, the earth is heaving with the dead, not buried deep but almost ready to break the surface. He estimates that there may have been 20,000 deaths each year in Roman Britain, making 4 million buried persons in total from the period, '& consequently so great a number of urnes dispersed through the land as may still satisfie the curiosity of succeeding times and arise unto all ages'.

All ages? I wonder if there are more fragments to be found. I am encouraged by Browne's assurance that among these urns were 'none above 3 quarters of a yard in the ground'. Is there a chance that some remains lie so shallow still?

The first challenge is to locate the site. Browne describes the field as 'lying between Buxton and Brampton, but belonging unto Brampton'; that is to say within the parish of Brampton. On my Ordnance Survey map, I trace the long and meandering parish boundary with a pencil. The urns were also 'not much more then a furlong from Oxned park'. I next mark a plausible limit for the park that once surrounded Oxnead Hall, and then draw a second perimeter a furlong out from this line. The place I am looking should lie just outside this line but still inside the Brampton parish line. There is indeed an area of overlap, luckily a small one. It is perhaps four or five hectares, a tiny parcel of land by the standards of modern East Anglian agriculture.

The site is easily surveyed from the embanked railway path that

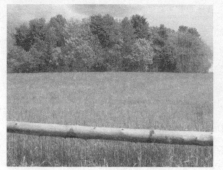

now bounds it to the south. Part of it is taken up with paddocks where some smart horses are grazing. On the far side, a strip plantation of pines blocks my view of Oxnead Hall. But most of it is still an arable field. Entry to the field is barred by a log with a PRIVATE NO ENTRY sign screwed to it. In addition, I'm aware the whole area is a scheduled archaeological site and that unauthorized excavations are not permitted.

At Oxnead, new owners are endeavouring to restore the hall to some of its former splendour. I have heard that their garden renovations have uncovered various artefacts, so one morning I extend my regular walk and knock on the door. I explain my Brownean project to the owner, and we discuss possible locations where Roman relics might lie. He happily shows me what has been found on his land: fragments of stoneware and Victorian medicine bottles and a perfect little flint axe head perhaps 5,000 years old. My appetite is whetted. He gives me the name of the farmer who tills the field I have identified, and the farmer kindly agrees to let me know when he will plough the stubble once the harvest is in. My plan is simply to follow his tractor. I reckon that its ploughshares dig in more than a foot, and there is a good chance they will turn up some long-buried fragments. I will not be doing any digging myself and so will not infringe any law.

When the call comes, though, I am abroad. On my return, I see that the field has not only been ploughed but also harrowed and drilled for winter barley. The autumn weather has been warm and wet, and fresh green spears are already coming up, made luminous by the low sun. My chance may be lost. I set off immediately, and start walking along the corrugated tracks left by the tractor. I am Browne's lop-sided badger running in the furrows. After half an hour or so, a pickup emerges from a track in the woods. It is Gary, who three years ago gave up his job as an electrician to become a farmer. His story is good to hear: we tend to hear only that people abandon farming. He tells me he often turns up pieces of pottery. At his home, he shows me a broken base in a cement-grey clay. He is not sure of its age, and nor am I. The pottery is thin and the rim line sharp; I assume it is recent, perhaps not much more than a century old. It reminds me I am more likely to find recent rubbish than Roman rubbish, and more likely to find Roman rubbish than Roman treasure.

Gary gives me a lift back to the field, and says I am welcome to see what I can find. I continue pacing along the tractor tracks, scanning right and left among the barley shoots for promising lumps. There are broken roots and fresh-faced shards of flint, indicating that the plough has cut deep. I find a few fragments of brick that could be from any period in history. After a short while, I spot a roughly square piece of caramel-coloured earthenware with arc-like creases on it that might just have been formed by mechanical turning. It is about a centimetre thick, but there's no glaze on it and no obvious ornamentation. Soon I come across a few more fragments. Two yellowish pieces are indubitably man-made. One, formed from two ropes of clay pressed together, looks like part of the curved handle of a large vessel. The other is part of the

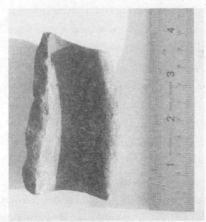

rim of a large pot. From the radius, I judge that the opening would have been almost a foot across. A curved lip runs along the rim, perhaps made for ease of carrying. After taking photographs, I replace the potsherds in the field where I found them, leaving sticks for markers in case I want to examine them again. I know that within a year they will be ploughed under once more, perhaps to lie buried for new centuries.

One hot summer's day, I make my way to Gressenhall, the former work-house where Norfolk County Council stores its archaeological records, to learn more about the Brampton urns. I am ushered into a room with a large table where I can spread out maps and photographs. I am the only visitor, and the heavy silence is relieved only by a bee buzzing in a ceramic jug somewhere on one of the shelves.

I am pleased to find that Browne is properly acknowledged as the first to have described the site, in 1667. There follows a long list of later investigations, a few in Victorian times, but commencing in earnest after the Second World War. Between 1964 and 1986, annual excavations uncovered evidence of a sizeable Roman town on the edge of the River Bure. Metal detectors have revealed many more Roman coins and other Roman artefacts, as well as the occasional object from other periods – a Bronze Age palstave, an Iron Age coin, a Saxon brooch.

The site was surveyed several times using aerial photography. The pictures taken during the long hot summer of 1976 are best. Then the soil shrank and the plants withered where they could not retain moisture, accentuating the contrast with areas that held more groundwater, such as buried ditches. These differences, called crop marks, only reveal their overall pattern when seen from the air. At Brampton, they show a large plot protected by a hexagonal perimeter of ditches. There are signs of a fort, a wharf on the river, a bathhouse and other amenities. On the road leading into the settlement, there are numerous small sites strung out like miniature versions of the sheds on a modern out-of-town indus-trial estate. They turn out to be kilns, 141 of them so far. The town was an industrial pottery, as Browne might in fact have logically concluded

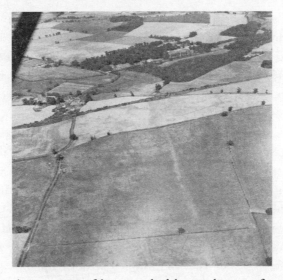

from the sheer variety of his pots, had he not been so fixated, after Walsingham, on funerary urns. His perforated cremation mausoleum was no more than a store for shelving fresh-made pots.

The bee's drone fills the room as I read on. No cemetery or burial site has been found in the town. In 1970, though, archaeologists found evidence of a cremation outside the bathhouse – a cremation jar 'upright with its rim level with the base of the plough'. Part of the rim was broken, presumably by the plough. It contained the bones of 'an adult, probably male, in the prime of life'; no grave goods.

Though he may have been mistaken in some of the conclusions he drew in the end from the relics uncovered at Walsingham and Brampton, Browne is nevertheless worthy of praise for his thorough method – describing, measuring, exhorting the workmen to proceed with care. It is an early sign of the shift that won't happen fully until the nineteenth century from the world of the antiquary reliant on providence, who treats ancient artefacts as curiosities, to the systematic archaeologist who is equipped to make scientific searches and can interpret objects with some understanding of the societies that created them.

*

Urne-Buriall has sometimes been taken as evidence that Browne himself was a melancholic, even that he suffered from what today we call depression. But I do not believe he was melancholic at all. Any melancholy is his literary affectation, appropriate to his subject here, and calibrated to the requirements of his market. It is never seen where he is writing without artifice, for example in his letters, where he can be as dull as anybody: 'I hope by Gods assistance you have been some weeks in Bourdeaux,' he writes to his son Tom in 1660. 'I was yesterday at Yarmouth...' And he goes on to discuss financial arrangements made for Tom's journey and to offer parental advice that any teenage travelling son would gaily ignore.

In the seventeenth century, melancholia occupied a broad middle ground of moods and mental states that ranged from what we now call depression to passing sadness. It was at once a condition, supposedly caused, like many diseases, by an imbalance of humours (specifically, an excess of black bile), and at the same time a behaviour. It could inhabit the body like a disease or it could be thrown on like a dark cloak. Gradually, the Latinate term 'melancholia' came to apply more exclusively to some of the more severe forms of depression, including conditions also characterized by delusions and violent behaviour, while the vernacular 'melancholy' was used for more bearable sadness, somewhat as we now distinguish between clinical depression and just feeling depressed. There were other stops on the line, too. The less fearsome acedia or accidie, for instance, was a state of mind related to the sin of sloth, a kind of torpor or laziness to which monks and scribes were said to be especially prone. Acedia was brought on by failure to fight off a demon, and unlike melancholia therefore carried with it an element of guilt.

We divide the spectrum of sorrows differently now, and these former distinctions have been lost to us. We jump from the unappealing solipsisms of low self-esteem, self-pity and worrying about our looks straight to what has recently been termed major depressive disorder. There is no acceptable middle ground. Major depressions are divided into further categories, of which the most remarked is the manic depression or bipolar

disorder that is sometimes exhibited by highly creative people. The association between creativity and mood swings was first noted by Aristotle
and then revived by the Medici's court philosopher Marsilio Ficino in
the fifteenth century, which may account for the aura of glamour that
then came to be associated with melancholia. 'It is somewhat ironic,'
observes the biologist Lewis Wolpert, who has suffered from depression,
'that in earlier times there was not always the stigma attached to depression that there is today, and that the melancholic thought of himself as
a rather superior being.'

There are other modern grades of depression, too – 'recurrent brief
depression', 'minor depressive disorder', and so on (I refer to the American *Diagnostic and Statistical Manual of Mental Disorders*). Aside from
these acute conditions, there is also dysthymia, a more persistent low
mood, and newer subsets of this such as 'seasonal affective disorder'. (It
occurs to me on a June afternoon when the temperature has struggled
to reach twelve degrees, and the wind has been pushing in off the still
cold North Sea a blanket of cloud unbroken for several days, that there
may even be a connection between the seventeenth-century vogue for
melancholia and the climate at that time of the Little Ice Age.)

This is all rather, well, clinical. How do I know if I am a melancholic in the seventeenth-century sense? Am I a melancholic if I fail to
respond positively to the overenthusiastic greeting of a cafe waiter, for
example? I was once dismissed from a job for having a 'bad attitude'.
Does that make me a melancholic? What if I go for a walk on my own?
Does that make me a melancholic? Perhaps it depends on the length
of the walk. These days, it seems that the wish to spend any time out
of the company of others is automatically suspect. To be absorbed in a
book is fast becoming another questionable activity. Yet these forms of
mental withdrawal can be revitalizing as well as symptomatic of mental
debilitation.

This very ambiguity is evoked by the brooding angel of Albrecht
Dürer's famous engraving *Melencolia I*. Initially, she appears as furious-
eyed, staring into the distance. As you look at her looking into the

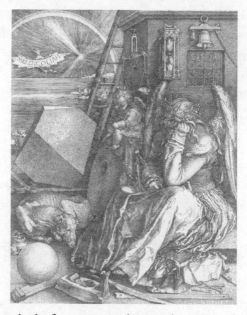

distance, though, the fury seems to abate; perhaps it is only pensiveness. Compass in hand, carpentry tools at her feet, it seems that her mind must in fact be productively occupied. But it is impossible to tell for sure. It is said that even the quantity of ink on different impressions of the engraving has affected our judgement: darker image, darker mood. And in any case, we no longer really know what we're talking about. 'For most of western European history, melancholy was a central cultural idea,' writes Jennifer Radden in her survey, *The Nature of Melancholy: From Aristotle to Kristeva*. 'Today, in contrast, it is an insignificant category, of little interest to medicine or psychology, and without explanatory or organizing vitality.'

Is it an insignificant category because nobody any longer behaves that way, or because we have stopped looking for it, or because we call it something else? Perhaps the world is so much improved that we have no call for melancholy. Turn it around. Did people in seventeenth-century England – and their physicians – believe they were experiencing an epidemic of melancholia? Was it a kind of contagion like the plague?

Was it something that fell within the normal range of emotional experience? Or was it simply a fashion? By 1733, noted the Bath physician George Cheyne, up to a quarter of the middle and upper classes were gripped by the 'English malady'.

Melancholia was prevalent enough to be labelled an English disease, but calling it a disease does not make it so, and it is equally hard to be sure whether we are experiencing a fresh outbreak today, or simply seeing a higher rate of diagnosis, or witnessing another passing fashion.

Now, back to my self-diagnosis. I suffer from acedia when I try to write; that is an occupational hazard. What makes me melancholic? Plenty: The inability of our civilization to rise above religious conflict. The inability of our civilization to take effective measures against climate change. Pygmy politicians. Apparently inexorably increasing social inequality. UKIP. The corruption of schools and universities by the ideology that their sole purpose is to equip people to fill 'jobs'. The ceaseless pandering to the lowest common denominator by the media. The orgy of mass-surveillance. The parlous state of the Norwich–London train service. The lengthening odds that Norwich City will remain in the ~~Premiership~~ Championship. My home's readiness to capitulate to the law of entropy. My garden, ditto.

I suffer from melancholia when I think of these things – although suffer is not quite the word, as there is also a luxury in feeling this way, a self-indulgent wallowing that is doubtless reprehensible, as I also do nothing, or can do nothing, about most of them. They are large and diffuse ills. Many are what we ironically acknowledge as 'first-world problems'. They offer no focal point for rage or action. Instead, they give me something to complain about, and who is to say this is not even a good, a point of connection with other people who feel the same way. We all like a good moan.

Now, what can we say about Thomas Browne's alleged melancholia? Around the age of thirty, he tells us in *Religio Medici*, he finds himself 'sometimes not without morosity'. Robert Burton begins *The Anatomy of Melancholy* with an exhaustive tabulation of all the possible causes of melancholy (it is really his way of warning his readers that he plans to write about everything). In Browne's case, we can rule out 'love-melancholy' (he would be happily married) and melancholy arising from physical diseases, 'In which the body works on the mind' (he never complained of anything more serious than deteriorating eyesight). We can rule out poverty, loss of liberty and dietary causes (he has admitted his tolerance of all foods). We can, I think, also eliminate causes 'Supernatural, As from God immediately, Or from the devil immediately, Or mediately, by magicians, witches.'

Natural causes might be more plausible, 'inward' ones, such as 'Old age, temperament' (Browne is fifty-two when he is writing *Urne-Buriall*), and 'Outward or adventitious' ones, such as 'Scoffs, calumnies, bitter jests', not to mention 'A heap of other accidents, death of friends, loss, etc,' all of which Browne indeed does feel acutely. Among causes of 'head melancholy', Burton lists 'Idleness, solitariness, or overmuch study, vehement labour, etc', and in regard to the last two of these we might also think Browne susceptible.

It is easy to find passages of text to support the idea that Browne was melancholic, both in *Religio Medici*, where as a vigorous, inquisitive young man he does 'conceive my selfe the miserablest person extant' were it not for the promise of death and another life, and especially in *Urne-Buriall*, where he writes: 'If we begin to die when we live, and long life be but a prolongation of death; our life is a sad composition; We live with death, and die not in a moment.'

There could have been a lot more death in *Urne-Buriall*. Browne writes it immediately following the years in which he and Dorothy lost five of their children. Their married life was one of 'unclouded happiness', as his biographer Edmund Gosse puts it. What can it be like, this happiness unclouded except by the deaths of five children? We have little conception now of how people pieced together their lives in the face of such routine tragedy. Death was expected at any time, and yet life must go on. People coped somehow, but this is not to say that grief over an individual loss was any less intense than it is for us now. One seventeenth-century definition calls melancholy 'grieving without suffi-cient cause'. But what is sufficient cause?

Browne might have written about his children's burials and described his feelings of loss. A noted contemporary, the Reverend Ralph Josselin, did just that in his diaries, with a candour surprising in a Calvin-ist clergyman (he recorded his feelings about everything else as well, including his thanks to God when he survives a bee sting on the nose). But Browne is more reserved, and after his marriage never writes again about his most personal emotions.

There are other things that make it easy to believe Browne might have had a melancholic tendency. As a physician, he was a witness to great suffering. He saw many patients die – although fewer, I like to think, than many of his fellow doctors. The medical profession today shows a high incidence of depressive illness, accords it a low priority, and makes it hard to seek help, according to recent research; there is no reason to think it was ever otherwise. In addition, Browne saw the country torn apart and its cultural treasures ransacked by the Civil War.

There are personal traits of character too. Modesty – Browne the man who wished to bid a total adieu to the world, remember – is a symptom. According to Freud: 'In grief, the world becomes poor and empty; in melancholia it is the ego itself.' Freud also noted that the melancholic has a keener eye for the truth than others; Browne surely has this. Even being a scientist can be construed as part of the problem. According to Ficino, 'for the pursuit of the sciences, especially the difficult ones, the soul must draw in upon itself from external things to internal as from the circumference to the center, and while it speculates, it must stay immovably at the very center (as I might say) of man.'

And of course Browne read a lot of books. And he wrote. Fairly or not, these activities have always been taken as signs of unhealthy intro-version and too much thinking.

But there are as many reasons to deny his melancholy. He was mentally alert. He was curious about everything, not unhealthily driven by one obsession, which is another chief manifestation of the melancholic character. He also fails to score as a melancholic just because he is getting old: 'many are too early old', he writes, thereby extracting himself from the mass, and assuring us of his evergreen virtues. He fails, too, by the definition of the poet Samuel Butler, who thought 'a melancholy man is one, that keeps the worst Company in the World, that is, his own; and tho' he be always falling out and quarrelling with himself, yet he has not power to endure any other Conversation.' Though uniquely proficient at quarrelling with himself, Browne also relished intellectual swordplay with others, and surely had little opportunity, in a house full of children and visiting patients, for solitude.

There is, besides, too much relish and good humour in his writing for melancholy to hold sway here. In *Urne-Buriall* he writes: 'the long habit of living indisposeth us for dying'. Joke, no? And just to be quite clear, he here and there puts himself on record as enjoying plays, music and laughter. It is significant that he does not say in *Religio Medici* that he is morose; he's 'not without morosity'. The litotes is a clue that we should not worry for him too much. He retains his equanimity through all his personal tragedies. 'Sense endureth no extremities, and sorrows destroy us or themselves.' Whatever his own sorrows, they certainly destroy themselves and not him.

*

The use of antidepressants has doubled in ten years in rich nations, including Britain and the United States, according to the Organisation for Economic Co-operation and Development. In Britain, usage trebled in the decade before that, the first full decade following approval of drugs such as fluoxetine, better known as Prozac, and the brightly named Lustral. There is evidence to suggest that the prescription and consumption of antidepressants has surged ahead of actual diagnosed cases of clinical depression.

Are people genuinely more depressed? Is the world fundamentally a more depressing place? It might be tempting to say so, but it seems hardly likely in the historical scheme of things. So are depression and its kindred sadnesses at last being recognized as true illness? Or is it that doctors are simply too ready, following the introduction of these drugs, to diagnose depression and prescribe antidepressants? The latter seems closer to the truth, if prescriptions are climbing faster than diagnoses. The drugs are filling a vacuum. It may not be easy to admit to suffering from a mental illness, but it is always possible to pop a pill, even if it has only a limited effect.

It is tempting to seek a description of depression in terms of chemical imbalances (how similar to humours!) that might then be subject to rectification by other chemicals in the form of drugs. If there are also psychological factors, then they are considered very much secondary (and neurological hardliners would retort that psychology is ultimately chemical, anyway). The chemical school has the upper hand. Mental behaviour is increasingly investigated by biochemical methods. This tends to make the behaviour less explicable rather than more so to ordinary people. It also reinforces the notion that the only way of altering that behaviour will be chemical. For example, animal experiments using pharmaceuticals may lead researchers to deduce associations between certain moods or behaviours and alterations in brain chemistry. This encourages an association to be made with similar signs in human patients and equivalent chemicals, which in turn produces an expectation that balance can best be restored by pharmaceutical means. This spiral from scientific study to medicalization is hard to escape, and quickly brings us to a point where depression of any degree, even normal grief or sadness, is to be regarded as chemically treatable and as an illness. (Consider the absurdity if we were to analyse normal happiness with the same intent.)

Drug therapies also raise the question of whether a patient is 'cured' in a way that psychological methods do not. 'Are patients who get better from depression really well?' was the title of a 2013 paper in the journal *Psychotherapy and Psychosomatics*. The German study compared acutely depressed and recurrently depressed subjects with a healthy control group, and found that even after treatment the recurrently depressed patients were seldom fully recovered. This suggests to me that while depression may be tackled with drugs, older, milder states of melancholia may yet persist, and need to be recognized and addressed in other ways.

Melancholia was medicalized in Thomas Browne's time, too. The standard remedy was St John's wort, which was also used to ward off evil, a reminder of the association of some forms of melancholy with invasion of the body by demons. St John's wort is still widely favoured in nature-loving Germany. In 2008, an analysis of clinical trials by the Cochrane Collaboration, the independent international assessor of medical trials, concluded that it was just as effective as modern drugs and produced fewer side effects. It has been approved by the British Medical and Healthcare Products Regulatory Agency but not by the American Food and Drug Administration, which favours pharmaceutical therapies.

In the United States and beyond, the modern equivalent of Burton's *Anatomy of Melancholy* is arguably the *Diagnostic and Statistical Manual of Mental Disorders* of the American Psychiatric Association. Its fifth edition (*DSM-5*) was published in 2013 amid passionate discussion of revisions made since the fourth edition of 1994. Much has changed in twenty years: there are new ideas about where and how to treat people, new pressures on families, hospitals and governments, and above all, new drugs. The *DSM* is a respected reference because it offers standardized definitions of mental disorders. These clearly aid diagnosis, if diagnosis means giving a condition an agreed name, and may lead to more appropriate treatment. Shared definitions are also important, as we saw with morgellons, in granting a legitimacy to conditions that may then fall clearly within the cover of health insurance policies. But they also imply single causes for particular moods, like the analogy of the single viruses that can give us measles or flu. This impression of neat duality lends further strength to the biochemical picture of mental disorder, at the expense of the messier psychological one, even though it is obvious that our environment – social, economic, even climatic – must play a large part in our mental health. However, few are interested in ultimate causes when there are drugs to treat present effects, and the *DSM* is no true catalogue of the tapestry of ways in which we all construe and misconstrue the world in which we find ourselves.

DSM-5 has redrawn a number of definitions so that some believe it to be medicalizing what was formerly regarded as no more than normal human behaviour. Dysthymia has been renamed 'persistent depressive disorder', for example. In some cases, single disorders have been split into two new disorders in order to avoid the appearance of over-diagnosis. The manual has followed recent psychiatric practice in splitting bipolar disorder into Bipolar I, for those who have experienced a full manic episode, and Bipolar II, for those who have not. But its most controversial move has been to draw within its ambit ordinary grief by dropping a so-called 'bereavement exclusion' included in the fourth edition, which served to excuse a period of depression lasting less than two months following the death of a loved one.

The beginnings of a link between grief and depression may lie with Freud's essay 'Mourning and Melancholia', written in 1915 at the height of the First World War, when there was much cause for both. Tackling the essentially subjective nature of melancholy, Freud cites Burton: 'the settled humor Burton describes as subject for treatment may merely manifest itself in more frequent occurrences of the "sad, sour, lumpish, solitary" feelings found, he says, in all men.' But if something is found in all men (and women?), it is by definition not a disease, just a part of the normal human condition. The advice in *DSM-5* is that six months is a normal period for grieving, although Professor David Kupfer, the task-force chairman for the manual, has conceded under pressure from critics that an individual's personal experience of grief might last 'two months, or a year, or years'. However, longer episodes of grieving are still liable to be re-categorized as disorders – 'prolonged grief disorder' or 'complicated grief disorder'.

Some psychiatrists have criticized these developments as the 'Americanization of mental illness'. They remind us that while depression of varying degrees of severity may be an effect of chemical imbalances in the brain, it is also a cultural construction, which has had and continues to have different meanings and interpretations in different times and places.

While acknowledging that true depression is a serious neurological condition, I believe that occasional bouts of melancholia are to be cherished as a proper response to the way we find the world. Exploring melancholy topics is a way to understand the serious reality of the world and to cope with it. It is not despair. The only alternative is childish denial.

It seems scarily easy to satisfy *DSM-5*'s diagnostic criteria for persistent depressive disorder or dysthymia when only two of the following six conditions need to be met: 'poor appetite or overeating; insomnia or hypersomnia; low energy or fatigue; low self-esteem; poor concentration or difficulty making decisions; feelings of hopelessness'. Even if the symptoms must present for most of the day, for more days than not, over a continuous period of two years, that still covers a lot of bases.

Of course, it is not possible to be normally melancholic all the time, just as it is not possible to be happy all the time. But a melancholic response can and should be just as legitimate as a joyful one. Certainly, my own melancholic feelings do not stop me finding joy elsewhere. Nor are they sufficiently dominant to qualify as depression; I know that these feelings, or feelings very like them, are shared, if not often communicated, by most people, and only some suffer from depression.

If finding no joy in life is one definition of depression – and this is the significance of the diagnostic emphasis on episode duration: how long are the periods when happiness is impossible? – then I am no depressive. Feelings of depression often centre on a significant loss, and neither have I a recent loss to report. I worry about losses in the abstract. Loss of biodiversity, for example, is undoubtedly a significant loss, but it is a loss that is not proximate or emotionally felt.

Nevertheless, I reserve the place of melancholy on the spectrum of emotions, and I reserve the right to feel melancholic as the mood takes me. What alternative response is there to an awareness of the cruelty of nature, or of man to man, or of the irreversible damage we are doing to the earth? These things are fixed. They do not call for an individual response; that would be impractical. Nor do they call for utter despair. It's just the way things are, or the way things are going, and that's a cause for sadness.

And yet this response is socially unacceptable. We pretend that melancholy does not exist. When we greet one another we are permitted to answer 'How are you?' only with 'I'm fine'. So many things conspire to distort our perception of the range of acceptable emotional response, from the relentless upbeat of the television presenter to the fake bonhomie of the corporate 'courtesy call'. Surely the right response to these falsities is a scowl and perhaps a curse. Anything less only encourages these travesties of human interaction.

The social pressure for positivity not only makes it hard for people who are depressed to say so; it makes it hard for any of us to speak truthfully about ourselves. A large area of our personal experience of the world is simply put beyond the bounds of decent discourse. If we cannot speak of sad things properly to one another, only one outlet is left: the couch. A major role of psychoanalysts today, according to Susie Orbach, is not even to relieve ordinary sorrow and despair but simply to provide 'recognition of the legitimacy of this kind of distress'. It cannot be healthy for society that we can only discuss this large part of our emotional experience by seeking professional help.

My potsherds provoke no outburst of melancholy in me. I am quietly satisfied to have found them with such a modest amateur effort. I heft them, rub the dirt from their crevices, and enjoy their weight and the muffled chinking noise they make as they settle in my hand. On the basis of the photographs I have taken, and information about where I found them, the Norfolk Museums and Archaeology Service has tentatively authenticated them as most likely Roman in origin. My pleasure at this is tempered by a rationalism that reminds me that these fragments, undecorated and unmarked as they are, in fact have very little to signify their belonging to any particular period to anybody but an expert. Without legends or decorations, signatures or fingerprints, I find it hard to summon a bond with the Roman-era potters.

Unlike Browne, who was there at the predawn of archaeology, I must assimilate my modest fragments with the far superior finds I have seen on display in public collections. It would be easy to feel jaded, exposed with such regularity to truly spectacular archaeological treasure in museums and on the dramatically orchestrated digs seen on television. But while my objects may not come complete with the polished display case and the knowledgeable caption, they do have something else. They are, I know, autochthonous: they have sprung from soil on which I have stood. For a few moments in the Brampton field, these fragments and I have shared a space that is not mediated by professional interpretation, and this is a rare thing. I am reminded, too, that this land was once common land, in the very act of enclosure when Browne was called here. These relics are common to us all.

I know that their involvement in funerary ceremonies is unlikely, and I am aware that I should not take the fact that these pieces were once underground as an indication that they were ever purposely or ritually put there. They are just bits of very ordinary pots. I wonder if Browne would have been disappointed to learn that the urns he found here had none of the melancholy significance that he presumed for them, and were merely utilitarian objects manufactured at the Brampton kilns to be taken down the river, perhaps to the coastal garrison at Burgh Castle or elsewhere in Roman East Anglia, where they would serve the mundane purpose of storing oil or wine.

I feel he would have taken it in good part. He was, after all, always ready to consider alternative answers to the problems presented by incomplete evidence. More than that, he was – unusually for his time, and unusually among his elite peer group – alert to the evidential importance of objects. For all his love of his library, he understood that there were times when things spoke more reliably than texts. An artefact from the ancient world, with all its mystery, was worth something that a scholarly source, perhaps much translated and transcribed, was not.

The word 'archaeology' at this time meant chiefly the study of ancient history through such written records. Browne therefore appears as a more modern kind of archaeologist, one who proceeds by direct observation and impartial description, in other words a scientist, albeit one still apt to leap to an extravagant conclusion if that will give him the pretext for imaginative digression. He even senses the potential – not to be realized for another 300 years – for forensic facial reconstruction. 'For since bones afford not only rectitude and stability, but figure unto the body,' he writes in *Urne-Buriall*, 'It is no impossible Physiognomy to conjecture at fleshy appendencies; and after what shape the muscles and carnous parts might hang in their full consistences.' He would surely have marvelled at modern archaeologists' success in regenerating the facial appearance of such figures from antiquity as Philip of Macedon, assembled from just three skull fragments, one of them containing a nick in it that was presumably made when he lost an eye to an Athenian arrow at the siege of Methone in 354 BCE. (I wonder, though, if he would have smelled a teleological rat in the recent regeneration from the skeleton found under a Leicester car park of the face of Richard III to such a close likeness of his known portraits.) He would have been astonished, too, at the DNA analysis of human remains, which were then, unless their identity was proclaimed by the urns that contained them, condemned to eternal anonymity, 'Not to be resolved by man, nor easily perhaps by spirits'.

The urns Browne has seen lack legible inscriptions, of course. The impossibility of knowing the former human identity of discovered bones is precisely what gives him such broad scope for his speculations. He describes these remains for readers who will appreciate that they are as such no more than 'Emblemes of mortall vanities; Antidotes against pride, vain-glory, and madding vices'.

How much less of a trace could we leave? Perhaps none at all is the ideal. I learn of a Swedish company that manufactures replica Roman burial urns ('approved by the Royal Navy') made of biodegradable unfired clay designed to dissolve into mud upon meeting with moisture in the soil. Way to go.

9
Objects

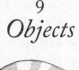

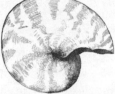

'Rarities of several kinds'

Musaeum Clausum

To tell Browne's story properly demands exhibits. What remains to us that is authentically his? Even the skull that I held is only a cast of the real thing rightfully reburied. There are manuscript copies of some of his books, there are letters. But I need things as well as words. Domestic things from his happy family household in the middle of Norwich. Curious things such as the plants and animals and pictures that inspired his writing. And urns.

Yes, where are the urns? The British Museum has a fine early Anglo-Saxon burial urn about the size of a watermelon, with an anthracite grey sheen and decorated with die marks and lines scratched in the clay, for which it provides this text: 'This handmade pottery urn (known as a Buckelurne) is similar to a group of fifty discovered by the physician Sir Thomas Browne (1605–82) in sandy soil less than three feet deep in a field near Walsingham in Norfolk.' But this specimen the museum admits was uncovered in Lincolnshire. So why drag in Browne? And where are the fifty?

The Norfolk Museums and Archaeology Service has catalogued the finds made over the years at both the sites Browne wrote about, the

Walsingham of *Urne-Buriall* and Brampton, where he made his later note on the same topic. I recall that I was prohibited from taking the pieces I found there because it is a registered archaeological site. The Norfolk archaeological staff were quite stern about this when I merely floated the idea that I might go looking. Surely the older, more complete urns have been carefully preserved. Where are Browne's urns? I ask Tim Pestell, the senior curator of archaeology at Norwich Castle Museum. His reply is swift and negative: 'unfortunately this is not known and we don't have any ourselves'.

What of Browne's own effects? His main house in Norwich was demolished in 1842 to make way for a bank and later for the building that now accommodates Pret a Manger. The drawing room contained

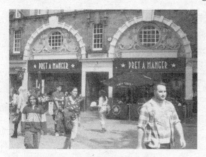

an imposing oak overmantel, the only part of the house that was salvaged. It was carved with the coat of arms of James I flanked by caryatids and large onyx bosses. It is easy to imagine such a thing as the focal point of the household, with the family gath-ered round a generous fire. His so-called garden house, an older building just around the corner from the main house (the one on the site now occupied by the Primark store), eventually fell into disrepair and was demolished in 1961. Here, a fancy plaster ceiling and a door were rescued from the skip. I read in a Festschrift produced to mark the tercentenary of Browne's death in 1982 that the ceiling is held in storage by Norwich council, while the door is supposedly on display at the Strangers' Hall Museum in the city.

Browne's collection of scientific and antiquarian objects has been even more effectively scattered. It is not known what he kept in his cabinet of curiosities, which was undoubtedly less of a cabinet and more like the whole of his house and garden. But it is certain, from the admiring comments of John Evelyn, who had seen more than a few such collections, that it was a good one. Browne's will – perhaps the only really dull piece of writing he ever produced – does not specify individual curiosities, but merely leaves to his wife Dorothy all his 'plate Jewells and all my goods whatsoever lowly'. It seems likely that the best of the curiosities would have gone to Browne's only surviving son, Edward, with whom he corresponded so entertainingly on the keeping of ostriches and such matters, since he also inherited Thomas's library of more than 2,000 volumes. The books were auctioned a few years after Edward's death in 1708, but it is not known what happened to any collection of objects.

We can surmise many of the items that Thomas Browne cherished, either in specific detail or in general outline, from his writing and especially from his descriptions of his own experiments undertaken to establish the truth behind a vulgar error. There would have been preserved birds – perhaps the kingfishers and bitterns, the stork and the roller that we encountered earlier – and the skulls and skeletons of Norfolk animals kept for purposes of anatomical comparison as well as for their natural

beauty. There would have been stones with unusual properties such as the eagle stone, a standard item in many cabinets of curiosities. Birds' eggs would recall Browne's investigations in embryology. There would be other minerals, chemicals, instruments and apparatus. Among these more or less expected items are sure to be a few more fantastical things, such as the horror that Browne fashioned out of fish skins, imitating the example of Ulisse Aldrovandi, who demon-strated how the 'Hieroglyphical fansie' that is the cockatrice – a creature supposed to have the head,

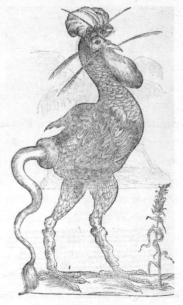

wings and feet of a cock and the tail of a serpent – might be fraudulently assembled out of 'Thornbacks, Scaits, or Maids' (all kinds of ray, fish whose thick, tapering tails no doubt passed very nicely for serpents').

The probable richness of Browne's collection of objects may be guessed at from the variety of his books, which skip easily between natural and cultural history, ancient and modern writers, fictions and purported fact, reading for education and reading for amusement. His Greek and Roman volumes include plays (both tragedies and comedies) and the stories of Homer and Virgil, as well as works of philosophy and classical science such as Plato's *Timaeus* and Aristotle's selected works. Some of these books promisingly blur boundaries: Pliny the Elder's *Natural History*, the august source of so many vulgar errors; Ovid's *Metamorphoses*, with its moral tales of shape-shifted humans. Others display Browne's need to be informed even about subjects he hardly touched upon in his own writing: Vitruvius on architecture, and an introduction to music by the Norwich composer Thomas Morley.

There is contemporary literature, too: Milton, Spenser, Jonson, and George Herbert's extraordinary devotional collection *The Temple*, in which many of the poems are typeset to resemble features of ecclesiastical architecture. He has Pascal's *Pensées*, but not, it seems, Montaigne's *Essais*, with which his own candid and questioning writing is so often compared. His theological reading includes works of conventional devotion by Augustine of Hippo, Jerome, and Thomas Aquinas, as well as the satires of Joseph Hall, the Bishop of Norwich, a Calvinist who could nevertheless record with moving regret the Puritan destruction of the treasures of his cathedral during the Commonwealth. But there are also philosophical enquiries that dare to question the existence of God.

Browne's medical library includes the essential ancients, the Greek Hippocrates and Roman Galen, and is augmented by the works of the Renaissance physicians who had built the reputations of the universities where Browne studied, principal among them the Padua anatomists Vesalius, Fabricius, Falloppio and Realdo Colombo. He kept up to date with developments in his professional field, adding new works by his fellow Padua alumnus William Harvey on the circulation of blood and the development of animals, as well as by a rising generation of home-grown medical innovators, such as Francis Glisson, the first to describe rickets, Thomas Willis, who made strides in the anatomy of the brain and nervous system, and Thomas Sydenham, 'the English Hippocrates'.

Some of his most thumbed books are the natural histories, especially the several volumes of Aldrovandi, as well as Pierre Belon on birds and Guillaume Rondelet on fishes. Later he adds the catalogues of English plants produced by John Ray, the taxonomist who first defined the concept of species in nature. In other fields of science, he has William Gilbert's *De Magnete*, Galileo's *Dialogue Concerning the Two Chief World Systems* and other works, and Isaac Barrow's edition of Euclid's *Elements*. For his atlas, he has a modern edition of Mercator, but it is already in need of revision. There are more edgy works, too, such as the alchemical treatises of Paracelsus, Basil Valentine and Michael Sendivogius, whose esoteric obsessions cannot quite disguise the emerging principles of systematic chemistry. It is a fast-changing world. Later acquisitions demonstrate the turn to a more systematic experimental science than he cared to consider for his own distraction: Francis Bacon, René Descartes, Robert Hooke, and *Some Considerations Touching the Usefulness of Experimental Naturall Philosophy* by Robert Boyle, who elucidated the concept of pressure in gases.

Browne also has a copy of *Difficiles Nugae*, by Sir Matthew Hale, the judge in the Bury witch trial, an exploration of the same sort of phenomena investigated by Hooke and Boyle that the distinguished jurist produced in the 1670s, hoping belatedly to confound the modern scientists and to find in these mysteries not a materialist explanation but evidence of spiritual causation. It is not good science. What is Browne doing with it? I like to think that he was given it by Hale, seeking approbation for his eccentric theories, and that he accepted it out of politeness and quietly put it on his shelves unread.

Browne has, finally, a small number of catalogues of works assembled by some of the great collectors: the German Jesuit Athanasius Kircher;

Elias Ashmole, who catalogued and was later deeded the collection of John Tradescant, which he augmented with his own objects to form the basis of what would become the Ashmolean Museum in Oxford; and the Danish physicians Ole Worm and Thomas Bartholin, who introduced a new Nordic exoticism to cabinets of curiosities. The glorious illustrated frontispiece to Worm's *Museum Wormianum*, for example, includes a kayak, a stuffed polar bear hanging from the ceiling, and a narwhal tusk propped up in the window.

A local perspective on curiosities comes from a magnificent painting known as *The Paston Treasure*. It shows some of the prize possessions of the Pastons, which Browne would have seen on his visits to the family as a friend and physician. The picture appears unexpectedly as an illustration, offered without further comment, in a chapter of John Berger's famous book *Ways of Seeing* about the display of wealth in art. But it was not just a display of wealth. Robert Phillips, another friend of Sir William Paston, wrote to him in 1658: 'You have exceeded all others of our nation that have been famous in their collections...Your museum abounding with an infinite variety of the most choice and admired rarities.' This private 'museum' was housed at Oxnead Hall, the Paston seat

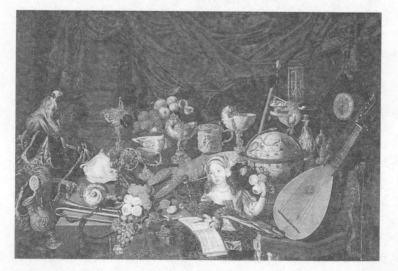

since 1597, where it was matched by an outdoor 'cabinet de verdure', a rectangle of planted beds with raised walkways from which one could look down on the growing specimens as if they too were exhibits in a display case.

Painted some time in the 1670s by an unknown Dutch artist, *The Paston Treasure* shows the kind of objects that were typically acquired by the well heeled and well travelled in the seventeenth century. Sir William ventured as far as Egypt and the Holy Land, while his son Robert became one of the original fellows of the Royal Society. Among the items they choose to display are a tobacco pipe sourced from the Virginia colony, fine porcelain from China, nautilus shells on gold stands, intricately engraved cowries, an enamel and gold pocket watch, a lute, viol, sackbut and other musical instruments, a large cooked lobster and abundant fruit. A globe is turned to show us that the Pacific Ocean and Mexico are the latest territories to be mapped, but the California coastline is still conjecture. A vervet monkey perches on the shoulder of a handsome black slave boy. Sinking beneath this sea of high-class jumble is a little girl who might almost be a discarded doll; she is Mary Paston, who was shortly to die of smallpox. An hourglass, an extinguished candle and various timepieces serve as symbols of mortality.

Browne's collection was certainly less ostentatious and more 'curious' than his rich client's. But it is likely also that it was less disciplined and less well stocked than the cabinets of Aldrovandi or Kircher or Worm. What is the point of these cabinets of curiosities? Their contents are curious and their owners are curious too, often in both senses of the word. They are collected not for instruction; that would come later, with the emergence of modern scientific disciplines and taxonomy. They only begin to set out some of the boundaries that will be observed by modern museums regarding what belongs to an overall order, and what is miscellany, what belongs to legitimate scientific enquiry, and what to whimsy. They are instead chaotic and heterogeneous, and that is part of the point. The display is not so much of objects, single or curated as a collection, but of the richness of the mind that has assembled them. This comes across in the variety, the unexpected juxtapositions, and above all the crammedness into spaces that seem like the cranial interior itself. These days, of course, we are able to project this jumbled interior vision into the ether with the minimum of effort via Pinterest or Tumblr. Instagram even offers visual filters that enable users to give their images an air of antiquity like a collection gathering dust.

The seventeenth century was a time of sharp wits, and the collectors, often idle as well as rich, found themselves the butt of jokes. John Donne satirized the collecting habit. But the most focused attack came from Thomas Shadwell in his play *The Virtuoso*, whose protagonist Sir Nicholas Gimcrack enthusiastically imitates the serious experiments of Hooke and Boyle, only to come up with absurd results. Perhaps the scientists' real imitators, such as Hale, were among Shadwell's targets, too: at one point in the play, Gimcrack announces that he is bottling air, not in order to analyse its substance, but in an effort to capture the spirit of the places where it was bottled. In 1710, the *Tatler* magazine extended the joke, publishing a letter purportedly written by Gimcrack's widow in which she tries to dispose of her husband's collection: 'If you know any one that has an Occasion for a Parcel of dry'd Spiders, I will sell them a Pennyworth.' Dorothy Browne must have faced the same predicament when Thomas died.

These satirical attacks seem to have had a quite an effect on proper science. During the 1670s and 1680s, the membership and income of the Royal Society fell back after the initial rush of members following its foundation in 1660 under the patronage of the restored king. Was it the lampooned silliness of the society's projects that put off new scholars, though, or in fact their very seriousness that put off gentlemen in search of lighter amusement?

Science is far less embattled today, whatever some of its pulpiteers would have us believe. People understand that it does not always deliver breakthroughs, and they perhaps even dimly appreciate why it is important that science does not punish 'failure' in the way that other fields of human endeavour so often do. Science is able to withstand what little mockery it receives, and has even institutionalized the satirical process in the form of the alternative Nobel Prizes, known as the IgNobel awards. Winners in 2013 included a Japanese team for 'assessing the effect of listening to opera on mice which have had heart transplants', and a pair of archaeologists who ate a shrew in order to see what would happen to its bones in the human digestive system.

In the crueller climate of a few hundred years ago, it was sometimes wiser to imagine collections than to assemble them in reality. In virtual space, serious intent and parody could run side by side. In *Pantagruel*, for example, Rabelais, one-time lecturer in medicine at Montpellier, mocks the growing scholarly literature by proposing a few titles of his own: *On the Art of Discreetly Farting in Company*, *Of Peas and Bacon, with a Commentary*, *The Mumblings of Celestine Padres*, and so on, 'Some of which are already in print'. Very different indeed is Francis Bacon's *New Atlantis*, which, in the guise of a voyage to an unknown island, presents a wish list of earnestly desired practical innovations: new alloys, deep freezes, solar-powered skyscrapers, animal-testing laboratories, and open-access publishing of research. But both works are united by the entirely hypothetical nature of their content.

Browne's short tract *Musaeum Clausum or Bibliotheca Abscondita* (The Barred Museum or The Flown Library, let's say) is another such work. It operates on several levels. First, it is an effective rebuttal to the satirists, being a more subtle and erudite satire than theirs. Penned by the collector Browne, it is therefore an exercise in self-mockery. But it also functions contrarily as a practical defence of the keeping of curiosities. For the items in Browne's imaginary cabinet are not opulent gewgaws or obsessively decorated nothings. They may have a point. Some of the entries in *Musaeum Clausum* form a kind of addendum to *Pseudodoxia Epidemica*, being evidential pieces that would serve, if they existed, to dispel a vulgar error. For example, Browne tells us, in Aldrovandi's cabinet of curiosities housed at the Senate of Bologna, 'there was preserved in Glass a Cub taken out of a Bear perfectly formed, and compleat in every part'. He mentions this foetus in order to refute the popular myth that mother bears literally lick their cubs into shape, a belief that may originate in the fact that bears give birth to proportionally the smallest young of all the mammals. We no longer believe this, of course, but we retain the expression 'to lick into shape'. Other exhibits might be summoned as material evidence against fraudulent practices in medicine: once you can point to a narwhal tusk, for example, it is easier to see off quacks who claim to have cures based on ground unicorn horn.

Finally, and unexpectedly, many of the 'exhibits' in *Musaeum Clausum* are not clever jokes or factual points of reference but speculative desiderata entirely in accord with Baconian thinking. They are emblematic of knowledge lost or knowledge yet to be obtained that would advance the state of natural philosophy. This is an entirely legitimate mode of scientific thinking, which is echoed in contemporary science by books such as *What Remains to Be Discovered*, by the long-serving editor of *Nature*, John Maddox, and John Brockman's compilation of scientists' answers to the question, 'What do you believe is true, even though you cannot prove it', published as *What We Believe But Cannot Prove*. Between them, they encompass everything from yet smaller subatomic particles to explain the unsatisfactory set we have now to the discovery of faster-than-light travel and extraterrestrial life.

Browne presents *Musaeum Clausum* in a letter to a now unknown recipient as 'a Collection, which I may justly say you have not seen before'. It carries the subtitle *containing some remarkable Books, Antiquities, Pictures and Rarities of several kinds, scarce or never seen by any man now living*. He lists two or three dozen each of books, pictures and artefacts in sufficiently pedantic detail that it is possible to believe they may actually exist. If the whole collection could be assembled, it would make a splendidly distracting exhibition in a public gallery.

The catalogue sets out various types of work that might for one reason or another have evaded conventional collection: notable works known to be missing, imagined works by notable writers, replacements for lost and stolen manuscripts, superior versions of slight works by well-known authors of whom better had been expected, and well-known works executed alternatively by different authors. Apart from works that would sate a literary curiosity, Browne also wishes to see documentary proof of historical events that will answer unanswered questions or furnish evidence that a certain shadowy event in history was definitively resolved one way or the other. He would like to see accounts of historical events by persons better qualified to comment than those who did happen to be there. And to see missing halves of correspondence, and to read the thoughts of great philosophers and scientists on some of the problems they never got round to tackling. In painting, he envisions landscapes of terrain where artists seldom go, portraits offering evidence of claimed resemblance of one person to another, and pictures to prove that certain unlikely historical events really happened.

These are some of the categories that Browne identifies, but his intent – at once earnest and mischievous – is best shown by example.

> A punctual relation of *Hannibal*'s march out of *Spain* into *Italy*, and far more particular than that of *Livy*, where about he passed the River *Rhodanus* or *Rhosne*; at what place he crossed the *Isura* or *L'isere*; ... at what place he passed the *Alpes*, what Vinegar he used, and where he obtained such a quantity to break and calcine the Rocks made hot with Fire.

> A Fragment of *Pythaeas* that ancient Traveller of *Marseille*; which we suspect not to be spurious, because, in the description of the Northern Countries, we find that passage of *Pythaeas* mentioned by *Strabo*, that all the Air beyond *Thule* is thick, condensed and gellied, looking just like Sea Lungs [i.e. jellyfish].

> An exact account of the Life and Death of *Avicenna* confirming the account of his Death by taking nine Clysters together in a fit of the Colick; and not as *Marius* the Italian Poet delivereth, by being broken upon the Wheel...

Perhaps, though, these fanciful paragraphs don't rise up off the page for us quite as they did for Browne's learned reader. A word or two of commentary may assist.

> The Letter of *Quintus Cicero*, which he wrote in answer to that of his Brother *Marcus Tullius*, desiring of him an account of *Britany*, wherein are described the Country, State and Manners of the Britains of that Age.

In September 54 BCE, Cicero had written to his brother accompanying Julius Caesar's expedition: 'You, however, I can see, have a splendid subject for description, topography, natural features of things and places, manners, races, battles, your commander himself – what themes for your pen!' Quintus either did not reply or his letter was lost. Such a description would be the first written account of the British Isles, antedating by some 150 years the brief sketch of Tacitus in his *Agricola*. As such, it presumably would have offered a description of the natives of Britain before they had lost their innocence, as it were, and fell under the influence of their Roman conquerors.

> An Ancient British Herbal, or description of divers Plants of this Island, observed by that famous physician *Scribonius Largus*, when he attended the Emperour *Claudius* in his Expedition into *Britany*.

A desirable might-have-been, as there is no indication such a work was ever produced, by Scribonius Largus or anybody else. Any work that brought together classical medical scholarship and the medicinal plants native to Browne's land would be of more than academic interest to him.

> A Sub Marine Herbal, describing the several Vegetables found on the Rocks, Hills, Valley, Meadows at the bottom of the Sea, with many sorts of Alga, Fucus, Quercus, Polygonum, Gramens and others not yet described.

What a wonderful idea. Do we have it yet? Browne is scientifically visionary enough to see that medicines might be extracted from marine vegetation, although he follows the misleading supposition of his time that each marine species must be the analogue of a terrestrial plant. John Gerard's famous *Herbal* contains woodcuts of 'sea oke or wrack', 'hairy river-weed' and other aquatic plants depicted through wavy lines to give an underwater effect. But this and later works only include a token few marine plants among their more exhaustive lists of land plants. More than three hundred years later, there is still no submarine herbal. Such catalogues of the earth's biodiversity gain poignancy now because we know we are driving species to extinction even before we have been able to list them. Many of those marine plants we do know are meanwhile being subjected to intensive study by 'bioprospectors' looking for novel molecular substructures around which to design new pharmaceuticals.

Among paintings Browne wishes to see are:

> A Moon Piece...A delineation of the great Fair of Almachara in Arabia, which, to avoid the great heat of the Sun, is kept in the Night, and by the light of the Moon

> A Snow Piece, of Land and Trees covered with Snow and Ice, and Mountains of Ice floating in the Sea, with Bears, Seals, Foxes and Variety of rare Fowls upon them

> Large *Submarine* Pieces, well delineating the bottom of the Mediterranean Sea, the **Prerie** or large Sea-meadow upon the Coast of *Provence*, the Coral Fishing, the gathering of Sponges, the Mountains, Valleys and Desarts, the Subterraneous Vents and Passages at the bottom of that Sea ...

❦❦❦❦❦❦❦❦❦❦ ❦ ❦ ❦❦❦❦❦❦❦❦❦❦

prairie (*Miscellany Tracts*, 1684): This is the first adoption into English of the Old French word *praierie*. It did not catch on, there being few tracts of land of sufficient size in England to warrant it, even in Norfolk. H. L. Mencken suggests that it did not travel on to England's colonies in the New World either, but instead entered American usage separately through French Canada some time before the American Revolution, along with such typically American words as 'chowder', 'depot' and 'bureau'.

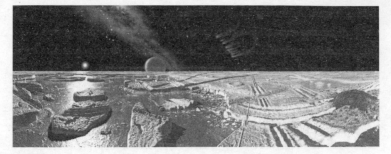

These seldom attempted artists' subjects are still rarities. They have their logical extension today in landscape paintings of unvisited planets. The doyen of this admittedly recherché genre was Chesley Bonestell, who illustrated popular books about space exploration and created artwork for films such as *War of the Worlds* and *Cat-Women of the Moon*. The work of successors, such as Jon Lomberg, who produced illustrations for Carl Sagan, is now informed by scientific data from the planets, which enables more accurate representation of features such as the colour of the sky, but these canvases remain above all imaginative visions, suggesting real places that people might one day visit. This makes them direct descendants of the 'American sublime' paintings of the nineteenth century – grand, empty landscapes commissioned with the aim of encouraging people to settle out west, often executed by artists who had themselves ventured no further than, say, Pennsylvania.

> Some Pieces *A la ventura*, or Rare Chance Pieces, either drawn at random, and happening to be like some person, or drawn for some and happening to be more like another; while the Face, mistaken by the Painter, proves a tolerable Picture of one he never saw.

Browne might have enjoyed Louis Tussaud's House of Wax at Great Yarmouth, a museum of waxworks described as the world's worst when it closed in 2012. Their Adolf Hitler looks like Hugh Bonneville, and Diana, Princess of Wales, looks like a transvestite. Some memorably bad 'photofit' likenesses made by police artists have nevertheless proved their worth. In 2006, an Australian cartoonist, Bill Green, foiled an attempted burglary at his home, and then produced an instant caricature which enabled police to identify the man and apprehend him minutes later.

A Commentary of *Galen* upon the Plague of *Athens* described by *Thucydides*.

Thucydides was an accurate reporter, but no physician. He gives a memorable description of the symptoms – he was infected himself – but not sufficient to identify the cause of the disease that struck Athens in 430 BCE. It is unlikely that Galen, who would not come on the scene for another 600 years, would have got much further. In 2006, DNA analysis of human remains from an excavated cemetery indicated the presence of typhoid fever, although other causes have not been ruled out.

Spirits and Salt of *Sargasso* made in the Western Ocean covered with that Vegetable; excellent against the Scurvy.

Occasionally in his list, Browne conceives of something that would be of practical use, such as this medicine, capable of being made at sea, for the treatment of scurvy, which was at the time a great affliction to mariners. Sargassum algae are today under investigation as a possible medium for the absorption of dissolved heavy metal pollutants such as cadmium.

A fair English Lady drawn *Al Negro*, or in the Æthiopian hue excelling the original White and Red Beauty, with this Subscription, *Sed quandam volo nocte Nigriorem*.

In 1993, the Hungarian-American designer Tibor Kalman reproduced a photograph of Queen Elizabeth II digitally manipulated to appear '*Al Negro*' in a race-themed issue of *Colors* magazine, a promotional publication of the fashion retailer Benetton. The image was greeted with mock consternation by the popular press in Britain. Science has been unable to establish whether, as the Latin epigram of Martial here quoted would have it, a man who is offered a willing white girl is really more desirous of one black as night.

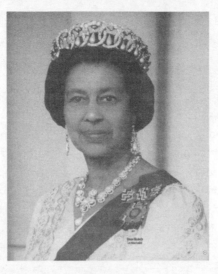

A large ostridges Egg, whereon is neatly and fully wrought that
famous battel of Alcazar, in which three Kings lost their lives,
[and also that parody of *The Iliad*] the Homerican Battel between
Frogs and Mice, neatly described upon the Chizel Bone of a large
Pike's Jaw

Our banal equivalent today of these examples of extreme crafts-
manship are those corporation logos carved out in single atoms. In
1989, IBM scientists used a scanning tunnelling microscope to position
thirty-five atoms of the element xenon to spell out the company initials.
In 2009, Stanford University physicists surpassed what might seem to
be the ultimate limit of one bit of information per atom when they used
a technique called electronic quantum holography to create the initials
S U in interference patterns less than an atom's width across. It is disap-
pointing that the creators of these small miracles are content merely to
produce advertisements for their employers.

Pyxis Pandorae, or a Box which held the *Unguentum Pestiferum*, which
by anointing the Garments of several persons begat the great and
horrible Plague of *Milan*.

Today, phials of the only known stocks of the smallpox virus are preserved by research centres in the United States and the Russian Federation, ostensibly for use in the development of improved vaccines and antiviral drug treatments, following the otherwise total eradication of the disease declared by the World Health Organization in 1980.

The ease with which such parallels may be drawn leads me to wonder whether somebody somewhere does not even now have plans to open a real *Musaeum Clausum* that will be able to truly surprise us, jaded as we are by the endless supply of performing kittens and spoof public announcements on the Internet, with more solid horrors and wonders.

The Strangers' Hall Museum turns out to be less intriguing than it sounds. It is a miscellaneous collection of fixtures and fittings from old Norwich houses displayed in the residence of the Tudor mayor who made the decision to admit the Dutch and Walloon 'strangers' to the life of the city in the 1530s. He gave some of these migrant workers rooms under his own roof. Perhaps one day a caravan used as accommodation by Eastern European vegetable pickers will be similarly preserved.

I find the door said to have come from Thomas Browne's garden house, a heavy oak affair of four panels, ill fitting in its Tudor frame. In the transom panels above the door is carved the date 1570 and some ornamental growth that looks like artichoke plants. But the object has no caption and, as I learn when I enquire, no provenance. There is nothing to say it came from Browne's house at all. The knowledge that it did – if knowledge it was in 1982 – has become ignorance.

Of the plaster ceiling and the Jacobean overmantel there is not even this possible sighting. The Norfolk Museums and Archaeology Service comes back to me to say it has no location record for either object. In short, the county appears to have destroyed or mislaid everything materially connected with Browne: his houses, his gardens, the urns, the lot. Is this astonishing negligence or forgivable wastage? I am disturbed at the losses, of course, but I cannot deny a creeping Brownean satisfaction that these precious things have disappeared, perhaps to be dug up – metaphorically or literally – at who knows what future date. I can only echo Browne, signing off *Musaeum Clausum*: 'He who knows where all this Treasure is, is a great *Apollo*. I'm sure I am not He.'

From time to time, Norwich's arts bodies remind themselves of their duty to commemorate Browne with what little material they can find. Such an occasion arises as I am working on this book. *Curiosity: Art and the Pleasures of Knowing* is a touring exhibition organized by the Hayward Gallery in London of things that artists have found curious, or have made so. It includes many of the expected items: a narwhal tusk, Albrecht Dürer's *Rhinoceros*, and Robert Hooke's *Micrographia*, opened to the page where there is a fabulous engraving of a flea as big as a cat. The fragile glass models of fragile sea creatures made by the Bohemian father and son Leopold and Rudolf Blaschka share space with Nina Katchadourian's apocalyptic montages made on long-distance flights by spilling rockfalls of complimentary nuts across the glossy travel scenes in seat-pocket magazines.

For its Norwich appearance, the curators have affectionately added in a homage to the city's famous curioso. The cast of his skull is here, a familiar friend. The fair manuscript edition of *Religio Medici* that I once held is open so that all may admire Browne's decorous handwriting. A random assortment of bladder stones alludes to Browne's medical career, and to the fact that he may have suffered from bladder stones himself. The curator Brian Dillon explains Browne's inclusion. 'He's an increasingly important figure for people looking at the way the arts and sciences come together,' he tells me. I am cheered that Browne's star is felt to be on the rise again.

In a splendid fractal recursion, *Curiosity* also features a large architectural drawing of an imaginary museum in which are displayed all the objects I have just seen, dreamily transformed in scale and re-hung in grand new spaces. It is the work of the artist Pablo Bronstein. I search the Beaux Arts galleries for the drawing in the drawing but do not see it. Of course, Browne's bits and pieces are not there either.

What sticks in my memory, though, is not this work or the narwhal

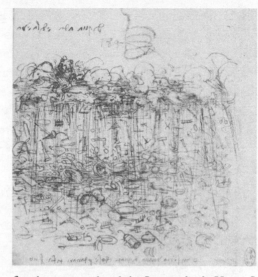

tusk or the flea, but a tiny sketch by Leonardo da Vinci. Somebody at some time has given it the title 'A Cloudburst of Material Possessions', and it does indeed show a rain of consumer products from the early sixteenth century – combs, bellows, bowls, even a pair of compasses are hammering down from the sky. It is on loan from the Royal Collection. I wonder what the Queen makes of it.

It leads me to wonder again about the meaning of objects, the value we attach to them, and how that value changes over time. What does it really matter that a few of the things that once cluttered Browne's life appear to have been lost?

To the person who buys or makes or finds an object, there is always an associated memory, of a place, or an occasion, or of some personal exchange, that gives it meaning. The thing alone means nothing. My Brampton potsherds convey their meaning to me chiefly because they play a part in my Brownean quest. Without that quest, they might conceivably hold some lesser value because they link time and place in a way that appeals to me, reminding me that there was once a thriving Romano-British community in my neighbourhood. But whatever their value, it is related entirely to my making an association.

This memorial weight cannot be felt by others, however much they try. They must make their own associations. Even our own parents' photographs from the time before we were born are almost meaningless to us. Shorn of this meaning, objects become nothing more than substitutes for something else, generalized signs of lost personal significance, tangible markers of something else that should be there or that we would like to recover. Their presence marks a greater absence.

I do not know what Browne felt about consumer possessions, but I do know what he felt about books. Surprisingly, he thinks there are already too many in the world. He would see whole libraries perish if it meant that he could hold some authentic older fragment, such as 'the perished leaves of *Solomon*'.

Few people keep a cabinet of curiosities today, but we collect like never before. We do so largely because we can. Our consumer society has so arranged it that we can afford more and more things. We buy because we seek comfort and security in our lives, and because we want something to pass on to the next generation. We hope that something we owned becomes something of what we were.

We are beginning not only to keep more than we have a use for but more than we even have room for. Instead of keeping our possessions around us, we now put them in remote storage facilities. According to the Self Storage Association, the United Kingdom has 30 million square feet of rentable storage space, as much as in the whole of the rest of Europe, but still only one-fifteenth of the space available in the United States. Not only are these locations proliferating, but people are leaving their stuff in them for longer. Our homes are becoming the galleries for the temporary exhibition of our lives, while the permanent collection resides in a tin box on the edge of town. We have become nomadic hoarders, an oxymoron accurately expressive of our societal inability to strike a balance between things and experiences, the comfort of possessions and the excitement of events.

This cannot go on for ever, or the whole countryside will be as full of our unregarded treasures as Browne once imagined the earth to be of the bones of all the departed generations. It seems not a moment too soon, then, that we are also exhorted to join an equally new trend – to declutter. Spontaneously throwing out large amounts of what we have accumulated may be read as a decisive rejection of the culture of consumerism. A good clear-out also implies a moral cleansing. But this may be a deceptive view. It may not be that easy to reverse the Pavlovian training of centuries suddenly to accept that happiness comes of getting rid of stuff rather than acquiring it. After all, each decluttering clears space for a new cluttering.

This is not only a consumer crisis. Museums quietly face the same dilemma, whether to keep on hoarding, or to let some things go. The rate at which archaeologists are unearthing human bones and artefacts now far exceeds the rate at which national collections can accommodate them. One solution is to keep records of new objects solely in digital form. But a more radical proposal calls for decluttering of existing collections on an institutional scale. The rule used to be that a find was kept unless there was a reason to throw it away. But, increasingly, there must be a reason to keep it, such as research or local community inter-est. At the Castle Museum Tim Pestell puts a local perspective on the problem: 'We have over 50,000 records of sites and finds in Norfolk, but we hold a tiny proportion of these in the museum.' Most objects, especially those found by metal detectors, are recorded and then given back to the finders. 'To give you some idea of the scale of this, we record over 20,000 finds per year in Norfolk, but only take in about quarter to half of one per cent of these to the museum per year.'

Even more discreetly, art galleries occasionally sell off works from their collections. They have a word for it that is seldom spoken aloud: deaccessioning. The procedure is considered ethical if the funds raised are used exclusively for the acquisition of new works that will raise the overall quality of the collection. But the business is still kept quiet, and the auction houses that do the dirty work are frequently instructed not to identify the consigner of a sale item. Some notable transgressions have come to light. In 2009, Southampton City Council caused a storm when it sold a number of paintings to raise money for a new museum dedicated to the *Titanic*. In 2013, the Museums Association threatened to withdraw membership from Croydon Council after it sold a collection of Chinese ceramics in order to raise funds to refurbish the borough's concert halls. The New-York Historical Society sold off nearly 200 'important old master paintings' in order to replenish its endowment – and reportedly to pay for new air-conditioning. Brandeis University in Waltham, Massachusetts, went a step further when it announced that it would sell off the entire collection of its Rose Art Museum in order to fund improvements in its teaching programme; only a lawsuit brought by museum board members prevented the sale from going ahead.

Why the fuss? Private collectors, after all, can freely sell off what they like, or rather don't like, and most galleries only have the space to display a tiny fraction of their collections. The underlying issue is usually to do with the public right of access to the work. But beneath that is a deeper fear that works of art may be destroyed altogether. If these institutions regard art as disposable to the extent of putting it up for sale, who is to say they are safe custodians of our culture?

In 2001, the artist Michael Landy probed some of these fears by getting rid of all his possessions, the process of reducing them to granules destined for landfill becoming an artwork called *Break Down*. More

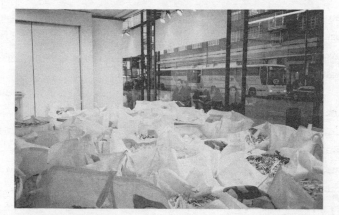

than 7,000 items were placed on a conveyor belt set up in an empty shop on Oxford Street, London's main shopping artery, and for two weeks Landy and his assistants disassembled and oversaw the destruction of each one. By the end, the artist was left with just an inventory and his memories.

I am keen to know how he felt about this unique exercise. We meet in the decidedly materialist setting of a fashionable private members' club in Shoreditch. Michael has a rugged, outdoor face and fixes me with an alert, steely eye. 'I'd never done a piece where people wanted to talk about it so much,' he tells me. The show brought out friends he hadn't seen for ages and the odd man with his possessions in a backpack seeking praise for his own load-shedding. His mother cried. 'It was like witnessing my own death,' Michael says. 'Possessing things partly makes us who we are.'

Landy began working up his nerve for the project by making the inventory and devising various schemes for the disposal. At first he thought he would just get rid of his consumer goods, but this rapidly expanded to include related personal items such as family photographs and his own and friends' artworks. The inventory is loosely organized by type (artworks, clothes, electrical and so on), but is thereafter in no particular order. What order could there be with items such as 'Brown Jonelle sunglasses with sand on them', '"Darth Vader" *Star Wars* badge',

- Certain romances of Robert Schumann destroyed by his wife Clara, composed in his later years of madness and melancholia, which may betray signs of the auditory hallucinations he was subject to; the eighth symphony which Jean Sibelius sent up his dining-room chimney in 1945 after nearly two decades' work on it.

- A transcript of the last speech given by President Abraham Lincoln of which it was said that it was so enthralling that nobody took down any note of it.

- A series of novels by Ian Fleming in the style of Sebastian Faulks, William Boyd and others who have exploited his James Bond character; and likewise by Jane Austen in the style of Joanna Trollope, P. D. James and others.

- The manuscript of Thomas Carlyle's account of the French Revolution burnt in error by John Stuart Mill's servant maid (to be displayed alongside the version rewritten from scratch that was finally published). Also, the superior version of T. E. Lawrence's *Seven Pillars of Wisdom* left at Reading railway station in 1919.

Verbatim accounts of some famous meetings:

— What Stanley really said to Livingstone

— What was the topic of conversation between Nelson Mandela + the Spice Girls

— The advice that Niels Bohr gave to Werner Heisenberg at their wartime meeting in Copenhagen

RECENT ACQUISITIONS:

Rachel Whiteread's <u>House</u> reassembled in the garden of the Tower Hamlets councillor who ordered the destruction of the original artwork.

Architectural drawings for a proposed Cuban missile site – as revealed by WIKILEAKS – the plans bearing a curious resemblance to the parts of a vacuum cleaner.

A commissioned Ordinance Survey map of Ambridge in Borsetshire, and not that substandard version produced by the BBC, which has neither scale nor contours.

The skeleton of the hamster eaten by Freddie Starr, as reported by the Sun newspaper in 1986 under the headline 'Freddie Starr Ate My Hamster', reassembled out of the bones of the animal recovered from the comedian's stool.

'THE BOYS' BIG BOOK OF UNKNOWN KNOWNS AND KNOWN UNKNOWNS'.
by Donald Rumsfeld
(FIRST EDITION)

MARBLE STATUE OF
EFF BEZOS, RECLINING
UDE, IN AMAZON
AREHOUSE No. 1,
ITH THE INSCRIPTION:
ooks are for nothing
t to inspire"
— EMERSON

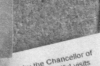

entire collection of high-visibility jackets worn by the Chancellor of
Exchequer, George Osborne, during four years of his dutiful visits
British factories.

An archive of all the images ever sent using Snapchat, indexed by user name and date for ease of use by parents and government agencies

'Single black cotton sock', 'Single tea bag' and 'Tesco Metro till receipt 30/4/00'? There were larger items, of course – chairs and televisions – and more sentimental ones, such as 'Jeff Koons flower dog fridge magnet from Guggenheim Museum' and 'Personal note for Gillian Wearing [now Landy's wife] from Michael Landy asking her not to leave towels on the floor'. Landy owned a brown sheepskin coat of his father's, and destroying that he felt would be 'a bit like disposing of my Dad'. In the event, though, he felt worse scraping the paint off a work by fellow artist Gary Hume under the eyes of the watching cameras.

And afterwards? 'I was euphoric for quite a long time, but at the same time I found I couldn't create anything.' The words of his one-time tutor Michael Craig-Martin stuck with him: 'It's an artwork, not a way of life.' Despite the title, it was not a sign of personal breakdown. Nor was it an utter rejection of worldly things, even though the artist's project was taken up by vicars as a subject for their sermons.

Then came the return to ordinary living. Michael realized he had made himself 'the perfect person to sell to'. Friends took him shopping, people sent him things in the post, and slowly he re-gathered a material existence. 'That was the discouraging part of it in a way. I'd had a beard trimmer, so I had to go and buy another beard trimmer.' He realized, too, that what he had been through was not a simple divestment but a more complex exchange. In destroying his possessions as a work of art, he had traded stuff for status. 'I became a much better known artist. That's the kind of messed up society we live in.'

How would Thomas Browne feel about the disappearance of the few objects by which we might have known him a little better? He would first of all probably be astounded that any of them survived for as long as they did. And then? I think he would have shrugged off the loss, recalling 'the slender and doubtfull respect I have always held unto Antiquities'. From time to time, Browne displays what we might now call intimations of entropy, the thermodynamic measure of order: he has a powerful sense of 'that power which subdueth all things unto it self' and of 'Time which antiquates Antiquities, and hath an art to make dust of all things'. He might have smiled at our difficulty in tracing his possessions as more nearly meeting his wish not to leave a trace upon the earth.

Browne collected not because he was covetous but because he was curious. His domestic trappings – the sort of thing that most appeals to our venal sensibilities today – are the very items likely to have interested him the least. Other objects he gathered were curious chiefly to him, and their interest might therefore be said to have died with him. Yet his overmantel and his ceiling are already a lot less interesting to me than these specimens without a record made of them (or if there were, it too has been lost). Would they have brought me closer to him? They might have. But I cannot know. Instead, I have been led into paths of speculation where I feel his spirit more strongly present.

10

The End

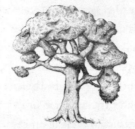

'A totall adieu of the world'

Religio Medici

THE VERY LAST chapter of the last of the seven books of *Pseudodoxia Epidemica* carries the heading: 'Of some Relations whose truth we feare'. After more than 200,000 words of heroic myth-busting, after all the puzzles of animals' habits and minerals' properties, after showers of wheat, and mermaids, and Adam's navel, Thomas Browne comes to a conclusion of arresting concern to the philosophy of science: that the truth is not always to be sought.

As there are many popular beliefs he is happy to refute and others that he cannot agree to, so here finally are some he heartily wishes would contain no truth. These are tales that reveal the horror of which humanity is capable. Browne's focus is not on episodes of mass-slaughter, but on heinous individual crimes, such as that of Rosamund, the Lombard queen who callously drinks from the skull of the father she has just had murdered. He fears there may be truth even in the story of Pygmalion, the sculptor who falls in love with the statue he has carved. Why? Because Herodotus has reports of Egyptian embalmers found engaging in necrophilia. Might not this infamous practice in fact be the origin of the myth? Browne is especially horrified by poisonings, such as the story of the monk said to have poisoned communion wine drunk by the Holy Roman Emperor Henry VII, who died suddenly in 1313.

Even if these awful things happened, they happened a long time ago. Why is Browne worried about them? It is because the very existence of an account of a crime may serve to put the idea into other men's heads. 'We desire no records of such enormities,' he writes. Evil acts recounted in this way may then be repeated and may come to be thought of not as the crimes they are but as unexceptional events. 'They omit of monstrosity as they fall from their rarity,' warns Browne. Better that we should be shocked afresh by each atrocity, which might then visit less often.

Browne's emphasis on poison is significant. It has metaphoric as well as literal potency: a poison may afflict the body politic as well as the human body. Poisoning is also a scientifically enabled method of killing. You don't need special knowledge to cut a man's throat, but you do if you are planning to poison him. This places those in the know – the technicians and the scientists – in a quandary. Should they withhold their knowledge? In cases like this, Browne thinks so. He praises the Roman physician Galen, 'who would not leave unto the world too subtile a Theory of Poysons', obliging would-be poisoners to make do with existing, ineffectual methods. 'In things of this nature silence commendeth history.'

It is not so much 'what you don't know can't hurt you', as 'what you don't know you cannot use to hurt yourself or others'.

Now, what should be our attitude to deadly knowledge in these days when the moral question is vastly magnified by the destructive powers at hand and by the rapidity with which information may spread? Do we withhold that knowledge? Can we? Who are 'we' in this transaction, and who are 'we' then withholding from? Or is the reverse course of action better, to disseminate the knowledge and trust people to exercise their own moral judgement about using it?

For there have certainly been recent cases of the kind that Browne fears where news of one horror has inspired others to commit similar horrors. The Bridgend area of South Wales saw at least nine suicides in 2007, three times the annual average. In the years that followed, the suicide rate remained abnormally high. By 2012, there had been seventy-nine fatalities, mostly young adults, mostly by hanging. It was acknowledged that there had been a cluster effect – not simply a high incidence of unrelated events – in which reporting in the news and on social media had prompted copycat episodes. The phenomenon is not entirely new: the publication of Goethe's *The Sorrows of Young Werther* in 1774 is also said to have prompted a wave of suicides in imitation of the eponymous disappointed lover. But it does have the potential to be made much more dangerous by modern media.

A month to the day after the Columbine High School shooting in Colorado in April 1999, in which two student assailants shot dead twelve pupils and a teacher, another American high school student, in Georgia, took a gun to school and shot six fellow students. The gunman had chosen the date as significant. The Columbine perpetrators had been influenced in their turn, it seems, by the Oklahoma City bombing of 1995. People have the right to know about such dreadful events, of course. But is it conceivable that a way of reporting on them might be devised that would inspire fewer feats of emulation?

And what of the larger stories whose truth we fear today: the world-enshrouding hazards of climate change, crises of supply in food, water and energy, pandemic disease and nuclear war, the familiar horsemen of our particular apocalypse? Our difficulty here is not so much that the truth is out there and adding to the danger we face, or that it is effectively withheld from us – although it undoubtedly is in some of these cases – but that we find it hard to gauge an appropriate response when presented with what information there is. In the case of climate change, we receive abundant scientific warnings but consistently fail to take adequate measures in response. The actual danger may be deliberately underplayed, possibly because governments in possession of the information to assess the dangers do not have an effective response to them.

Dire warnings are in any case easy to ignore when the end of the world tends not to arrive. Living 'in this setting part of time', Browne fully expects the world to end quite soon, although for him this is nothing to be feared. He is confident that it will not be brought about by natural calamity or human actions, however. 'I beleeve the world growes neare its end, yet is neither old nor decayed, nor will ever perish upon the ruines of its owne principles,' he writes. For a moment he nevertheless imagines what a purely physical end of all things might be like, asking: 'Whether if the motion of the Heavens should cease a while, all things would instantly perish?' What would become of the heat, the light and the ethereal 'influence' on which we depend? But he sets the question aside: it is too presumptuous to be thinking of such forces not under God's control. The end he has in mind will be divinely wrought.

It seems this is still the ending that many would prefer. In 2011, a radio network in Los Angeles announced that Judgement Day would fall on Saturday 21 May of that year. The evangelical preacher Harold Camping predicted that the Rapture would be accompanied by fire, earthquakes and five months of slow dying for those unlucky souls not spontaneously raised to heaven.

Camping's coup de théâtre offers a timely case study in the power of credulity. For the more publicly you take a stance, the harder it is to admit later you were wrong. As it happens, a film crew making a documentary about belief was on hand to witness people's reactions. The cameras observed how some looked at Camping's 'evidence' and started to believe in what he was saying. Once embarked on this path, these followers found, the only respectable course open to them was to deepen their belief. The emotional investment involved was often high. Some of Camping's flock fell out with their families. A few quit their jobs rather than have to explain why they would not be coming in to work on the Monday following the Apocalypse. Taking these irrevocable steps, they became more and more convinced of the rightness of their chosen path. As the fateful day approached, they watched for signs – mainly on television. On Thursday the 19th, Camping took to the airwaves, still confident that his timing was right. He and his followers now found that they themselves were news. When on the 21st would it happen?

the media wanted to know. What would happen to them? What would happen to everyone else?

The Saturday came and went. The film-makers packed away their kit and discreetly left in the early hours of the next morning. On the 22nd, Camping appeared genuinely bewildered when doorstepped by reporters. He called a press conference to repeat that he had been right about the date, and that a spiritual Rapture had occurred, but that the physical Rapture would now take place on a new date of 21 October. The rescheduled Rapture would be a humane affair and quickly over. 'Probably there will be no pain suffered by anyone because of their rebellion against God,' a chastened Camping told the press.

As Camping's position shifted from apparently genuine bafflement that the end had not come as he had predicted to one of perhaps cynical calculation as to what to do next, his followers began to feel released from their obligation to uphold what they had believed. Support for Camping's ministry collapsed – although not, of course, before many of them had donated large sums of money to his cause.

As it happens, Camping met his maker in December 2013, but he is unlikely to be the last of his kind. Opinion polls routinely find that nearly half of American Christians expect Jesus to return within fifty years – the kind of interval that people perhaps feel equates to an expected remaining lifetime, the kind of interval that Thomas Browne perhaps had in mind too, although he wisely refrained from ever predicting a date.

However great the thrill of anticipation, our true end story is not likely to be an abrupt cataclysm. It will be something more gradual contained in the ever-changing myths we carry with us. What we now call climate change our successors will doubtless rework into a story of greater human resilience to 'natural' disasters. Likewise, our *story* of biodiversity is not the profile of sharp decline in many species that the data indicate; the human lifespan is not long enough to convince ourselves of this. It is instead based on the constant habit of celebrating what we see around us, in other words, what we've still got, even though what we've still got is so much less than earlier generations celebrated in their time. Eventually these stories recede into deeper mythology. They become the dodo, the Great Plague of London, the Black Death, Noah's flood.

It is because of science that we know what we do about the dangers before us. In some cases, scientific knowledge makes us aware of a danger we would not easily sense, such as the depletion of the ozone layer. In others, it enables us to recalibrate unreasonable fears. This is the case, for example, with the danger that our planet faces from a strike by an asteroid, where an improved ability to track 'near-earth objects' has led astronomers to downgrade expectations of a damaging impact. These are both hazards about which Thomas Browne of course knew nothing.

It seems obvious, then, that our scientific knowledge ought to be put to use in determining how we should live. Rather than fear the truth, we should seek it out and use it to shape society, say the statisticians and scientists who are the leading advocates of what has come to be known as evidence-based policy. Browne's cri de cœur finds itself at odds with the recommendation for policy to be based more closely on scientific evidence. There is science that we ought to suppress, he believes.

The concept of evidence-based policy is an extension of evidence-based medicine, which is a reaction against the popularity of alternative treatments such as homoeopathy for which there is no evidence base of medical effectiveness. Its central tenet is that policies should only be adopted if they have been tested and shown to work. Aside from the obvious desire to produce demonstrable change for the better, evidence-based policy is driven by a wish to overcome the futile shuttling between policies irrationally shaped by opposing political ideologies. Policies would be informed no longer by data-poor political rhetoric, but by the results of randomized control trials like those used in the development of pharmaceuticals. By greater reliance on solid data, the argument goes, we will free ourselves from unexpected and unwelcome outcomes.

But there are problems. One of the greatest is the anti-democratic sensibility that lurks behind demands for evidence-led government. In

The Geek Manifesto, Mark Henderson berates those who do not choose the scientific path, but succumb instead 'to the postbag effect', seeming not to understand that it is one of the duties of elected politicians to respond to the views of their constituents. This form of scientific authoritarianism may work – in terms of achieving objectives more effectively than the messy system we enjoy at present – but it is not a form of government that has much time for ordinary people. Already, it is notable, for instance, how many evidence-based policy initiatives – from imposing drinking curfews to banning homoeopathy – would lead to curtailments of individual freedoms. Moreover, excessive reliance on evidence may lead to a situation where politicians no longer dare to argue for what they think is right out of pure moral conviction.

What role should scientific evidence then play in our lives? When should it be heeded? Are there times when it should be ignored? In the end, it does not much matter that our politicians are largely ignorant of science. It would be nice if they were not, of course. But it is more important that they know who they can turn to for reliable information when they need it, as is the case in other areas of policy. The evident truth (and let's extend this to include the use of data to project likely future scenarios) should not be feared, but nor should we always allow it to dictate the course of our actions.

In 1937, Winston Churchill wrote an article in the *News of the World* that ran under the headline 'Life in a World Controlled by the Scientists'. After some conjectures on the prospects for nuclear power, harmless recreational drugs, mind control, eugenics and robots, he comes to his point. Thanks to science, he says, we are gathering knowledge and power faster than virtues and wisdom. We have arrived at a condition where our power exceeds our intelligence and our intelligence outruns our 'nobility'.

It is, therefore, above all things, important that the moral philosophy and spiritual conceptions of men and nations should hold their own amid these formidable scientific evolutions. There are secrets too mysterious for man in his present state to know; secrets which once penetrated may be fatal to human happiness and glory. But the busy hands of the scientists are already fumbling with the keys of all the chambers hitherto forbidden to mankind. Without an equal growth of Mercy, Pity, Peace, and Love, Science herself may destroy all that makes human life majestic and tolerable.

Churchill's words might seem mere alarmism until we remember the date. He was talking about the influence of scientific innovation on government. Our dilemma today is to do with the influence of the scientific *method* on government. Would evidence-based policy lead to better outcomes? Are politicians equipped to implement it? Do they understand the meaning and value of scientific evidence? Do they know how to assess it? Can they be trusted not to twist it to their own political ends? And is the public ready for it? How is the voter to distinguish between a proposal that has evidence to back it up and the usual ideology?

An intelligent scepticism – scepticism, not cynicism – might seem to be part of the answer. But it is certainly not as simple as that. In 1987, Carl Sagan wrote that if scepticism were 'more generally available in American society', it might help to avoid national policies that only pretend to make us safe, while actually exposing us to greater danger. But the example he chose to illustrate his argument might now be used to refute him. He cited the Reagan administration's resistance to a comprehensive nuclear test ban treaty as a policy that no scientifically knowledgeable public would ever endorse. We know now that the Berlin Wall fell two years later. Who is to say that the apparently irrational policy option was not in fact the right one at the time?

I have chosen Thomas Browne to accompany me on this exploration of knowable and unknowable truth. He may seem an odd, even a perverse, companion to take. He is often wrong about things, and even when he is right, his scientific knowledge is bound to be out of date. But I have done it for good reasons: because I am fascinated by him, of course; because I am fascinated by his period; and above all because I believe the way he sees the world has lessons for us today.

I cannot extend Brownean scholarship. I have made no historical discovery about him, found no lost book, no forgotten manuscript (O happy author). Indeed all I seem to have found is that many of the objects supposed to have an association with Browne have disappeared. Nor can I offer the definitive interpretation of his texts (O naive author).

Instead, I hope I have found a way to bring Thomas Browne to wider notice. He deserves to be known beyond the groves of academe. It would be foolish to demand that he be given his rightful place. What is his rightful place? I would have him on the schools' national curriculum. But I could not claim that he is relevant – that dread word of Gradgrinds and purse-string holders everywhere. He is in many ways gloriously irrelevant. He is so different from the way we are now.

And yet he is the same. He is curious, he is fallible, he is doomy, he is hopeful. He is open-minded and at the same time resolutely wrong-headed. He is a contradiction, as we all are.

The seventeenth century was a time when science was only just beginning. Browne and his contemporaries knew they were standing at the start of something. If they ever envisioned the scientific project as a line in time, it would have been a line with its origin in classical antiquity and its end far into the indiscernible future (and quite probably some time after God had brought the world to an end). They would have positioned themselves on that line somewhere hardly advanced from the ancients. To be a scientist was not then a recognized professional activity, and yet what we now call scientific enquiry was surging ahead. So was everything else. Questions about the nature of the world were not walled off artificially from questions about the fabulous and fictional, the mystical and the numinous, which are also part of the world.

With the conveniently blurred vision of hindsight, we hail men like Hooke and Harvey as archetypal scientists in order to reinforce our own myths about the birth of modern science. They were among the first to experiment, to make sound observations, to draw logical conclusions. But they were also more complex – and, as we would find now, self-contradictory – figures than we allow. We imagine these men as systematic, disciplined observers. So they were. But this is not all they were. Newton was not only a genius in mathematics and physics, but also an adept in alchemy and magic. Yet this less respectable (to us now) side of his life was for a long time edited out of the standard heroic version. We fashion history to conform to the requirements of the present. And we struggle with the paradox of biography: you cannot tell the whole life. This has been especially so for the lives of scientists.

This is another reason for writing about Browne, a man whose misfortune it is to have fallen on the wrong side of the divide we have erected between legitimate scientific enquiry and unwarranted eccentricity. It is not his fault, nor is it the fault of his exquisite prose style. It is ours for erecting the divide in the first place. A curioso might ask about all things.

Thomas Browne is a champion of the early modern period. But it feels to me as if we are only now standing at the threshold of an age that might deserve to be called early modern, if by 'modern' we mean the conscious rejection of the superstitious and irrational ways of the past, and the embrace of a life where scientific knowledge informs our progress in tandem with an appropriate humility.

Today's scientists see the same timeline of achievement, and imagine themselves…where along it? Further along, obviously. But how much further? They count many great discoveries and slide the marker confidently to the right. Answers have come. Some areas of science are perhaps nearing what might be called completion. Slide the marker farther along. Does the line have an end? Is it in sight? As we have seen further (by standing on the shoulders of giants), have we noticed also that the line is even longer than we thought? We glance back and see that the line now stretches far that way too. We know more than we used to. We know more than Browne knew. And we feel more certain about what it is that we know and what it is that we would like to find out next. We are sure that we no longer make the kinds of misjudgements he made. We are, aren't we?

I am looking out on my hated garden. The apple blossom is out and the birds are singing. I have just heard that storks are nesting in Norfolk for the first time in 600 years. Perhaps the new republic is not far behind. My quincunxial plantation waves gently in assent.

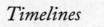

Timelines

1605

Born in London, 19 October.
Two weeks later, Guy Fawkes's
Gunpowder Plot is foiled. Religious
sectarianism will be a constant
presence in his life.

1611

1613

King James Bible

Montaigne's *Essays* appear in
English translation

1621

1623

Robert Burton,
The Anatomy of Melancholy

Shakespeare's First Folio
published

1620

English
Puritans land in
Massachusetts

294

1631–3 After Winchester and Oxford, he completes his medical training in the leading European centres, Montpellier, Padua and Leiden. He sees lived happily and unhappily by both Catholics and Protestants.

1635 He writes the *Religio Medici*: 'I teach my haggard and unreclaimed Reason to stoop unto the lure of Faith.'

1637 Is incorporated as a doctor of medicine. Settles in Norwich, England's second city, a thriving Hanseatic cosmopolis. He makes Norfolk his home. He watches its skies, trawls its waters, and pokes around in its soil. Here he finds life and death.

1641 Marries Dorothy Mileham. 'I could be content that we might procreate like trees, without conjunction, or that there were any way to perpetuate the world without this triviall and vulgar way of coition.' He gets over it. They have eleven children.

1626 Francis Bacon, father of the experimental method, dies, supposedly of a fever sustained while trying to preserve a chicken carcass by stuffing it with snow

1628 Charles I's physician William Harvey discovers the circulation of the blood

1633 Galileo forced to recant his belief in Copernican heliocentrism

1637 Descartes, *Discourse on Method*

1642–9 Civil War. He can see both sides. This is unusual.

1618–48 Thirty Years War intensifies with French entry against other European powers

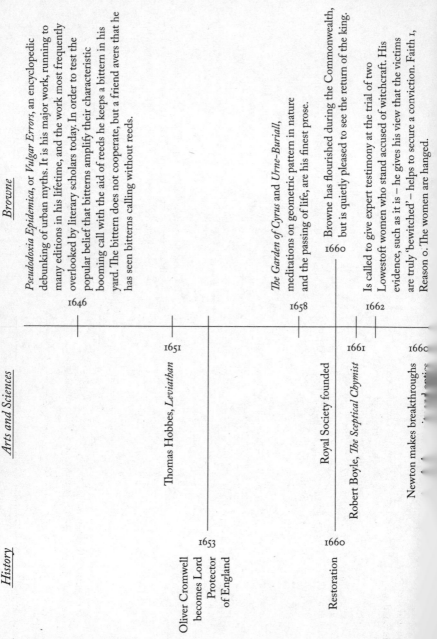

Browne

Pseudodoxia Epidemica, or Vulgar Errors, an encyclopedic debunking of urban myths. It is his major work, running to many editions in his lifetime, and the work most frequently overlooked by literary scholars today. In order to test the popular belief that bitterns amplify their characteristic booming call with the aid of reeds he keeps a bittern in his yard. The bittern does not cooperate, but a friend avers that he has seen bitterns calling without reeds.

1646

The Garden of Cyrus and *Urne-Buriall*, meditations on geometric pattern in nature and the passing of life, are his finest prose.

1658

1660 — Browne has flourished during the Commonwealth, but is quietly pleased to see the return of the king.

1662 — Is called to give expert testimony at the trial of two Lowestoft women who stand accused of witchcraft. His evidence, such as it is – he gives his view that the victims are truly 'bewitched' – helps to secure a conviction. Faith 1, Reason 0. The women are hanged.

Arts and Sciences

1651 — Thomas Hobbes, *Leviathan*

Royal Society founded

1661 — Robert Boyle, *The Sceptical Chymist*

1660 — Newton makes breakthroughs

History

1653 — Oliver Cromwell becomes Lord Protector of England

1660 — Restoration

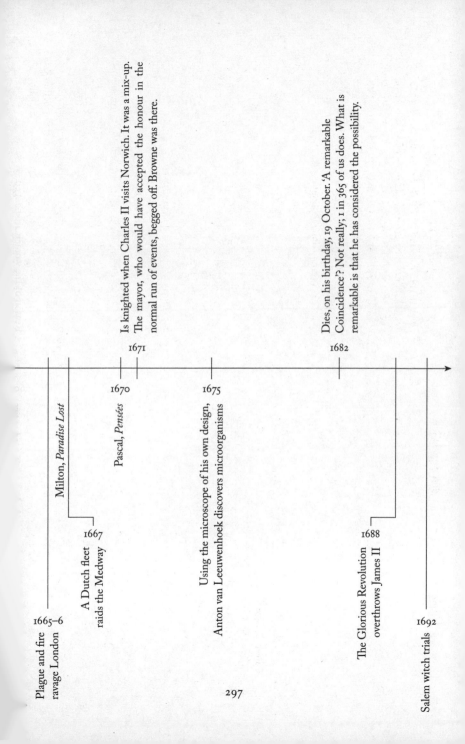

Plague and fire ravage London

1665–6

Milton, *Paradise Lost*

A Dutch fleet raids the Medway

1667

Pascal, *Pensées*

1670

Is knighted when Charles II visits Norwich. It was a mix-up. The mayor, who would have accepted the honour in the normal run of events, begged off. Browne was there.

1671

1675

Using the microscope of his own design, Anton van Leeuwenhoek discovers microorganisms

Dies, on his birthday, 19 October. 'A remarkable Coincidence'? Not really; 1 in 365 of us does. What is remarkable is that he has considered the possibility.

1682

The Glorious Revolution overthrows James II

1688

Salem witch trials

1692

297

Major Works of Thomas Browne

Religio Medici, 1643

Written soon after he qualified in the 1630s, and privately circulated before its authorized publication in 1643, *Religio Medici* is a highly personal confession and meditation on Christian faith addressed to those who might believe that, as a modern physician and scientist, Browne might have had no faith at all. 'I borrow not the rules of my religion from Rome or Geneva, but the dictates of my own reason,' he wrote. *Religio Medici* has been called the first celebrity autobiography. Like authors both earlier and later who dared to discuss religious belief from a rationalist standpoint, such as Galileo, Montaigne and David Hume, Browne's efforts were rewarded with a place on the papal index of forbidden books.

Pseudodoxia Epidemica, 1646

A vast catalogue of widely (epidemic) believed falsehoods (pseudodoxies), *Pseudodoxia Epidemica* is divided into categories animal, vegetable, mineral, human, pictorial, geographical, historical and biblical. Browne debunks many myths under each heading in richly varied ways, turning to ancient authority, transparent reason, or his own experimental demonstrations for persuasion. It was his most popular work, running into six editions during his lifetime.

The Garden of Cyrus, 1658

This is the most unusual and original of Browne's works and his most extended scientific speculation. Browne surveys many natural organisms, finding aspects of their shape, pattern and symmetry in common. He focuses especially on the significance of five-fold repetition in nature. His examples extend imaginatively but not always helpfully to human artifice. However, *The Garden of Cyrus* was conceived more in a spirit of play than with any serious numerological or cabbalistic intent.

Hydriotaphia, or Urne-Buriall, 1658

Browne's most celebrated work among scholars of English literature, *Urne-Buriall* contains his most high-flown and lyrical prose. He begins with a description of ancient funerary urns found in Norfolk and expands into a survey of the quintessentially human ritual treatment of the dead: 'Man is a noble animal, splendid in ashes and pompous in the grave.' The book concludes with a melancholic passage on the difficulties of knowing our ultimate fate: 'The long habit of living indisposeth us for dying.' *Urne-Buriall* was possibly intended as a companion work to *The Garden of Cyrus*.

Christian Morals, 1716

Written during the 1670s, but lost after his death, and published only in 1716, *Christian Morals* amplifies some of the ideas expressed in *Religio Medici* in seventy-nine short aphorisms, homilies and sermons. They are not exclusively Christian in tone and content, but offer broad advice as to how to live virtuously, embracing aspects of Aristotelianism, Epicureanism and stoicism as relevant to secular life as to a believer's. A specimen: 'Let thy Studies be free as thy Thoughts and Contemplations: but fly not only upon the wings of Imagination; Joyn Sense unto Reason, and Experiment unto Speculation, and so give life unto Embryon truths, and Verities yet in their Chaos.'

References and Further Reading

WRITINGS BY THOMAS BROWNE

Browne, Sir Thomas, *Notes and Letters on the Natural History of Norfolk*, ed. Thomas Southwell (London: Jarrold and Sons, 1902)

Keynes, Geoffrey, ed., *The Works of Sir Thomas Browne*, 2nd edn., 4 vols. (Chicago: University of Chicago Press, 1964)

Patrides, C. A. ed., *Sir Thomas Browne: The Major Works* (Harmondsworth: Penguin, 1977)

Wilkin, Simon, ed., *Sir Thomas Browne's Works*, 4 vols. (London: William Pickering, 1835–6)

British Library: Sloane 1847 MS

Norfolk Record Office: MS 21273; MS 212168

James Eason maintains an invaluable website containing most of Thomas Browne's writings at http://penelope.chicago.edu. The texts are the first editions of most works, but the sixth (and the last published during Browne's lifetime) edition of *Pseudodoxia Epidemica*.

My quotations from Browne's writings have been drawn from these sources, except in one or two instances where I indicate that I have quoted from different editions.

WRITINGS ABOUT THOMAS BROWNE

Barbour, Reid, and Preston, Claire, *Sir Thomas Browne: The World Proposed* (Oxford: Oxford University Press, 2008)

Barbour, Reid, *Sir Thomas Browne: A Life* (Oxford: Oxford University Press, 2013)

Batty Shaw, Anthony, *Sir Thomas Browne of Norwich* (Norwich: Browne 300 Committee and Jarrold & Sons Ltd, 1982)

Bennett, Joan, *Sir Thomas Browne: A Man of Achievement in Literature* (Cambridge: Cambridge University Press, 1962)

Browne 300 Committee, *Sir Thomas Browne, His Family and Friends: Catalogue of an Exhibition of Portraits and Memorabilia* (Norwich: Castle Museum, 1982)

Dunn, William P., *Sir Thomas Browne: A Study in Religious Philosophy* (Minneapolis: University of Minnesota Press, 1950)

Finch, Jeremiah S., *Sir Thomas Browne: A Doctor's Life of Science and Faith* (New York: Schuman, 1950)

Huntley, Frank, *Sir Thomas Browne: A Biographical and Critical Study* (Ann Arbor: University of Michigan Press, 1962)

Meyrick, F. J., 'Sir Thomas Browne: The Story of His Skull, His Wig, and His Coffin Plate', *British Medical Journal*, vol. 1 (1922) pp.725–6

Patrides, C. A., ed., *Sir Thomas Browne: The Major Works* (Harmondsworth: Penguin, 1977)

Post, Jonathan F. S., *Sir Thomas Browne* (Boston: Twayne, 1987)

Preston, Claire, *Thomas Browne and the Writing of Early Modern Science* (Cambridge: Cambridge University Press, 2005)

Whyte, Alexander, *Sir Thomas Browne: An Appreciation* (Edinburgh: Oliphant, Anderson and Ferrier, 1913)

Oxford English Dictionary, www.oed.com

Oxford Dictionary of National Biography, www.oxforddnb.com

Office of National Statistics, www.ons.gov.uk

INTRODUCTION

Borges, Jorge Luis, *Labyrinths* (London: Penguin, 2000)

Browne 300 Committee, *Sir Thomas Browne, His Family and Friends: Catalogue of an Exhibition of Portraits and Memorabilia* (Norwich: Castle Museum, 1982)

Browne, Sir Thomas, *La Religión de un Médico y el Enterramiento en Urnas*, trans. Javier Marías (Barcelona: Reino de Redonda, 2002)

Cushing, Harvey, *The Life of Sir William Osler*, vol. 2 (Oxford: Clarendon Press, 1925)

Dawkins, Richard, *A Devil's Chaplain* (London: Weidenfeld & Nicolson, 2003)

Forster, E. M., *The Celestial Omnibus and Other Stories* (London: Sidgwick & Jackson, 1911)

Gosse, Edmund, *Sir Thomas Browne* (London: Macmillan, 1905)

Gould, Stephen Jay, *The Mismeasure of Man* (London: Penguin, 1997)

Kushner, Tony, *Death and Taxes: Hydriotaphia and Other Plays* (New York: Theatre Communications Group, 2000)

Mackay, Charles, *Extraordinary Popular Delusions and the Madness of Crowds* (Ware: Wordsworth Editions, 1995)

Metcalf, Eleanor Melville, *Herman Melville: Cycle and Epicycle* (Cambridge: Harvard University Press, 1953)

'Mortal Remains', *Norwich Chronicle* (14 September 1840)

Nabokov, Vladimir, *Speak, Memory: An Autobiography Revisited* (London: Penguin, 2000)

Needham, Joseph, *The Great Amphibium: Four Lectures on the Position of Religion in a World Dominated by Science* (London: Student Christian Movement Press, 1931)

Norfolk Record Office PD 26/138

Ramsay, William, and Travers, Morris W., 'Argon and Its Companions', *Philosophical Transactions of the Royal Society A*, vol. 197 (1901) pp.47–89

Sagan, Carl, *The Demon-Haunted World: Science as a Candle in the Dark* (London: Headline, 1996)

Sebald, W. G., *The Rings of Saturn*, trans. Michael Hulse (London: Harvill, 1998)

Thompson, D'Arcy W., *On Growth and Form* (Cambridge: Cambridge University Press, 1961)

Tildesley, M. L., 'Sir Thomas Browne: His Skull, Portraits, and Ancestry', *Biometrika*, vol. 15 (1923) pp.1–76

Whalley, George, ed., *The Collected Works of Samuel Taylor Coleridge*, vol. 12 (London: Routledge & Kegan Paul, 1985)

Woodall, James, *Borges: A Life* (New York: Basic, 1996)

Woolf, Virginia, *The Common Reader* (New York: Harcourt Brace, 1925)

BIOGRAPHY

Ajdacic-Gross, V., et al., 'Death Has a Preference for Birthdays – An Analysis of Death Time Series', *Annals of Epidemiology*, vol. 22 (2012) pp.603–6

Brooks, Pamela, *Norwich: Stories of a City* (Ayr: Fort Publishing, 2003)

Browne, Philip, *The History of Norwich, from the Earliest Records to the Present Time* (Norwich: Bacon, Kinnebrook and Co., 1814)

Defoe, Daniel, *A Tour through the Whole Island of Great Britain* (Harmondsworth: Penguin, 1971)

Fuller, Thomas, *The History of the Worthies of England* (London: I. G. W. L. and W. G., 1662)

Hughes, Trevor, 'Sir Thomas Browne, Shibden Dale, and the Writing of Religio Medici', *Yorkshire History Quarterly*, vol. 5 (2000) pp.89–94

Hughes, Trevor, 'Sir Thomas Browne's Knighthood', *Norfolk Archaeology*, vol. 43 (1999) pp.326–31

Meeres, Frank, *Strangers: A History of Norwich's Incomers* (Norwich: Norwich HEART, 2012)

Phillips, D. P., Van Voorhees, C. A., and Ruth, T. E., 'The Birthday: Lifeline or Deadline?', *Psychosomatic Medicine*, vol. 54 (1992) pp.532–42

Phillips, David P., and Smith, Daniel G., 'Postponement of Death Until Symbolically Meaningful Occasions', *Journal of the American Medical Association*, vol. 263 (1990) pp.1947–51

Rawcliffe, Carole, and Wilson, Richard, eds., *Norwich since 1550* (London: Hambledon & London, 2004)

Reeve, Christopher, *Norwich: The Biography* (Stroud: Amberley, 2011)

Williams, Charles, 'The Will of Thomas Browne', *Proceedings of the Norfolk and Norwich Archaeological Society*, vol. 16 (1906) pp.132–46

Wrigley, E. A., and Schofield, Roger, *The Population History of England, 1541–1871: A Reconstruction* (Cambridge: Cambridge University Press, 1989)

Young, Donn C., and Hade, Erinn M., 'Holidays, Birthdays, and Postponement of Cancer Death', *Journal of the American Medical Association*, vol. 292 (2004) pp.3012–16

PHYSIC

Agnew, Jean, ed., *The Whirlpool of Misadventures: Letters of Robert Paston, First Earl of Yarmouth, 1663–1679* (Norwich: Norfolk Record Society vol. 76, 2012)

Arikha, Noga, *Passions and Tempers: A History of the Humours* (New York: Ecco, 2007)

Hunter, Michael C. W., and Davis, Edward B. eds., *The Works of Robert Boyle* (London: Pickering & Chatto, 2000)

Ernst, Edzard, 'Mistletoe as a Treatment for Cancer', *British Medical Journal*, vol. 333 (2006) pp.1282–3

Grell, Ole Peter, and Cunningham, Andrew, *Medicine and Religion in Enlightenment Europe* (Aldershot: Ashgate, 2007)

Hughes, J. T., 'The Medical Education of Sir Thomas Browne, a Seventeenth-Century Student at Montpellier, Padua, and Leiden', *Journal of Medical Biography*, vol. 9 (2001) pp.70–6

Hylwa, Sara A., et al., 'Delusional Infestation, Including Delusions of Parasitosis: Results of Histologic Examination of Skin Biopsy and Patient-Provided Skin Specimens', *Archives of Dermatology*, vol. 147 (2011) pp.1041–5

Kellett, C. E., 'Sir Thomas Browne and the disease called "the morgellons"', *Annals of Medical History*, vol. 7 (1935) pp.467–79

Loveday, Robert, and Loveday, Anthony, *Loveday's Letters Domestick and Forrein* (London: Nath. Brook, 1659)

Nagy, Doreen, *Popular Medicine in Seventeenth-Century England* (Bowling Green: Bowling Green State University Press, 1988)

Nuland, Sherwin B., *How We Die* (London: Chatto and Windus, 1994)

Pearson, Michele L., et al., 'Clinical, Epidemiologic, Histopathologic and Molecular Features of an Unexplained Dermopathy', *PLOS One*, vol. 7 (2012) e29908 doi:10.1371/journal.pone.0029908

Robles, David T., et al., 'Delusional Disorders in Dermatology: A Brief Review', *Dermatology Online Journal*, vol. 14 (6) (2008) p.2

Savely, Virginia R., Leitao, Mary M., and Stricker, Raphael B., 'The Mystery of Morgellons Disease: Infection or Delusion', *American Journal of Clinical Dermatology*, vol. 7 (1) (2006) pp.1–5

Schofield, Bertram, ed., *The Knyvett Letters, 1620–1644*, vol. 20 (Norwich: Norfolk Record Society, 1949)

Wear, Andrew, *Knowledge and Practice in English Medicine 1550–1680* (Cambridge: Cambridge University Press, 2000)

www.americanloons.blogspot.co.uk

ANIMALS

Clarke, M. R., 'Buoyancy Control as a Function of the Spermaceti Organ in the Sperm Whale', *Journal of the Marine Biological Association of the United Kingdom*, vol. 58 (1978) pp.27–71

Clarke, M. R., 'Function of the Spermaceti Organ of the Sperm Whale', *Nature*, vol. 228 (1970) pp.873–4

Forbes, Peter, *Dazzled and Deceived: Mimicry and Camouflage* (New Haven: Yale University Press, 2009)

Gould, Stephen Jay, *Wonderful Life: The Burgess Shale and the Nature of History* (New York: Norton, 1989)

Henderson, Caspar, *The Book of Barely Imagined Beings* (London: Granta, 2012)

Mabey, Richard, *Nature Cure* (London: Chatto & Windus, 2005)

Mills, Brett, 'The Animals Went in Two by Two: Heteronormativity in Television Wildlife Documentaries', *European Journal of Cultural Studies*, vol. 16 (2013) pp.100–14

Monbiot, George, *Feral: Searching for Enchantment on the Frontiers of Rewilding* (London: Allen Lane, 2013)

Mora, Camilo, Tittensor, Derek P., Adl, Sina, Simpson, Alastair G. B., and Worm, Boris, 'How Many Species Are There on Earth and in the Ocean?', *PLOS Biology*, vol. 9 (2011) pp.1–8

Schama, Simon, *The Embarrassment of Riches* (London: William Collins & Sons, 1987)

Taylor, Moss, and Marchant, John H., *The Norfolk Bird Atlas* (Thetford: British Trust for Ornithology, 2011)

www.memoproject.org

PLANTS

Bacon, Francis, *The Major Works*, ed. Brian Vickers (Oxford: Oxford University Press, 1996)

Ball, Philip, *The Self-Made Tapestry* (Oxford: Oxford University Press, 1999)

Batty Shaw, Anthony, 'Sir Thomas Browne's Meadow', *Notes and Queries*, vol. 18 (1971) pp.295–9

Coen, Enrico, *Cells to Civilizations: The Principles of Change that Shape Life* (Princeton: Princeton University Press, 2012)

Cooper, David E., *A Philosophy of Gardens* (Oxford: Clarendon, 2006)

Douady, S., and Couder Y., 'Phyllotaxis as a Physical Self-Organised Growth Process', *Journal of Theoretical Biology*, vol. 178 (1996) pp.255–312

Evelyn, John, *The Diary of John Evelyn*, ed. E. S. de Beer (London: Oxford University Press, 1959)

Hargittai, István, ed., *Fivefold Symmetry* (River Edge: World Scientific, 1992)

Lichtenfeld, Stephanie, Elliot, Andrew J., Maier, Markus A., and Pekrun, Reinhard, 'Fertile Green: Green Facilitates Creative Performance', *Personality and Social Psychology Bulletin*, vol. 38 (2012) pp.784–97

Luo, D., Carpenter, R., Vincent, C., Copsey, L., and Coen. E., 'Origin of Floral Asymmetry in Antirrhinum', *Nature*, vol. 383 (1996) pp.794–9

Rajchenbach, Jean, Clamond, Didier, and Leroux, Alphonse, 'Observation of Star-Shaped Surface Gravity Waves', *Physical Review Letters*, 110, 094502 (2013)

Sauret-Güeto, Susanna, Schiessl, Katharina, Bangham, Andrew, Sablowski, Robert, and Cocn, Enrico, 'JAGGED Controls Arabidopsis Petal Growth and Shape by Interacting with a Divergent Polarity Field', *PLOS Biology*, vol. 11 (4) (2013) e1001550

Stuart, Rory, *What Are Gardens For? Visiting, Experiencing and Thinking About Gardens* (London: Frances Lincoln, 2012)

Weyl, Hermann, *Symmetry* (Princeton: Princeton University Press, 1952)

SCIENCE

Ball, Philip, *Curiosity: How Science Became Interested in Everything* (London: Bodley Head, 2012)

Goldacre, Ben, *Bad Science* (London: Fourth Estate, 2008)

Henderson, Mark, *The Geek Manifesto* (London: Bantam, 2012)

Higby, Gregory J., 'Gold in Medicine: A Review of its Use in the West before 1900', *Gold Bulletin*, vol. 15 (1982) pp.130–40

Needham, Joseph, *A History of Embryology* (Cambridge: Cambridge University Press, 1934)

Pliny the Elder, *Natural History* (London: Penguin, 2004)

www.rsc.org/mpemba-competition/

TOLERANCE

A Tryal of Witches Held at Bury St Edmunds (London: William Shrewsbery, 1682)

Bostridge, Ian, *Witchcraft and Its Transformations c.1650–c.1750* (Oxford: Clarendon Press, 1997)

Bussein, Nathalie, *Breaking the Spell: Responding to Witchcraft Accusations against Children* (Geneva: UNHCR, 2011)

Evans, E. P., *The Criminal Prosecution and Capital Punishment of Animals* (London: William Heinemann, 1906)

Geis, Gilbert, and Bunn, Ivan, *A Trial of Witches: A Seventeenth-Century Witchcraft Prosecution* (London: Routledge, 1997)

Hale, Matthew, *Difficiles Nugae: Or, Observations Touching the Torricellian Experiment* (London: William Shrowsbury, 1674)

La Fontaine, J. S., *Speak of the Devil: Tales of Satanic Abuse in Contemporary England* (Cambridge: Cambridge University Press, 1998)

MacFarlane, Alan, *Witchcraft in Tudor and Stuart England* (London: Routledge, 1970)

Monmouth, Thomas of, *The Life and Miracles of St William of Norwich*, ed. Jessopp, A., and James, M. R. (Cambridge: Cambridge University Press, 1896)

Thomas, Keith, *Religion and the Decline of Magic: Studies in Popular Beliefs in Sixteenth and Seventeenth Century England* (London: Weidenfeld & Nicolson, 1971)

Witchcraft and Human Rights Information Network, *21st Century Witchcraft Accusations & Persecutions* (Lancaster: WHRIN, 2014)

FAITH

Dawkins, Richard, *A Devil's Chaplain* (London: Weidenfeld & Nicolson, 2003)

Dawkins, Richard, *The God Delusion* (London: Bantam, 2006)

Jones, Steve, 'When Science and Religion Mix', *Guardian* (31 May 2013)

Larson, Edward J., and Witham, Larry, 'Leading Scientists Still Reject God', *Nature*, vol. 394 (1998) p.313

Macaulay, Rose, *Some Religious Elements in English Literature* (London: L. and Virginia Woolf, 1931)

Pevsner, Nikolaus, *Norfolk 1: Norwich and North-East Norfolk* (Harmondsworth: Penguin, 1997)

Weaver, Warren, *A Great Age for Science* (New York: Alfred P. Sloan Foundation, 1961)

MELANCHOLY

American Psychiatric Association, *Diagnostic and Statistical Manual of Mental Disorders: DSM-5* (Washington DC: American Psychiatric Association, 2013)

Burton, Robert, *The Anatomy of Melancholy* (New York: New York Review of Books, 2001)

Center, Claudia, et al., 'Confronting Depression and Suicide in Physicians', *Journal of the American Medical Association*, vol. 289 (2003) pp.3161–6

Horwitz, Allan V., and Wakefield, Jerome C., *The Loss of Sadness: How Psychiatry Transformed Normal Sorrow into Depressive Disorder* (Oxford: Oxford University Press, 2007)

Orbach, Susie, 'The Sad Truth', *Royal Society of Arts Journal* (Spring 2012) pp.16–19

Radden, Jennifer, ed., *The Nature of Melancholy: From Aristotle to Kristeva* (Oxford: Oxford University Press, 2000)

Turner, Bryan S., *The Body and Society: Explorations in Social Theory*, 2nd edn. (London: Sage, 1996)

Wolpert, Lewis, *Malignant Sadness: The Anatomy of Depression* (London: Faber & Faber, 1999)

OBJECTS

Arnold, Ken, *Cabinets for the Curious: Looking Back at Early English Museums* (Aldershot: Ashgate, 2006)

Brockman, John, ed., *What We Believe But Cannot Prove* (London: Free Press, 2005)

Gerard, John, *The Herbal; or, Generall historie of Plantes* [new edn.] (London: Norton & Whittakers, 1636)

Landy, Michael, *Break Down* (London: Artangel, 2001)

Maddox, John, *What Remains to Be Discovered* (New York: Free Press, 1998)

Rabelais, François, *Gargantua and Pantagruel* (London: Penguin, 2006)

www.en.wikisource.org/wiki/Letters_to_his-brother_Quintus/2.15

www.improbable.com/ig/

THE END

Sagan, Carl, 'The Burden of Skepticism', *Skeptical Inquirer*, vol. 12 (1987) pp.38–46

Churchill, Winston S., 'Life in a World Controlled by the Scientists', *News of the World* (7 November 1937)

Illustration Credits

The author and publisher have made every effort to trace copyright holders. Please contact the publisher if you are aware of any omissions.

Illustrations with no credit indicated are © the author

Acknowledgements

It is said that the doctors where I live are in the habit of writing on certain of their patients' notes the abbreviation 'N4N', which stands for 'Normal for Norfolk'. I do not know if patients have a similar way of designating their doctors, but I can happily say that Dr Thomas Browne was never normal for Norfolk or anywhere else. He was, and remains, truly exceptional.

It has become apparent during the course of a project that has, one way or another, occupied me for the best part of a decade that many people quietly share my enthusiasm for this remarkable man. Others at least respected my passion for him even if they may have wondered whether I was quite normal as I asked to dig in their fields or through their archives or sought to establish the factual basis of some obscure piece of folklore.

Thanks go to the staff of the various Norwich museums and Norfolk county offices I visited, including Clare Agate, John Alban, Neil Alton, Catherine Blanshard, Giorgia Bottinelli, Jonathan Draper, Rosy Gray, David Gurney, Heather Hamilton, Belinda Kilduff, Susan Maddock, Hannah Maddox, Ian Palfrey, Tim Pestell, Helen Renton and John Renton.

Many other local friends and colleagues offered support and assistance, including David and Beverly Aspinall, Gary Bean, James and Evelyn Buchan, Marion Catlin, Enrico Coen, Matt Cooper, Charlotte Crawley, John Crane, Stephanie Douet, Kevin Faulkner, Krzysztof Fijalkowski, Chris Gribble, Christine Hood, Amanda Hopkinson, Claire and Sebastian Kokelaar, Henry Layte, Karen Lee, Vicky Manthorpe, Brett Mills, Gill Perficke, Keiron Pim, Alison Pressley, Elizabeth Purdy, Dominique Rey, Keith Roberts, Anthony Batty Shaw, Anthony and Ann Thwaite, Sarah Wilmot, Sheridan Winn.

Further inspiration and answers came from Vladeta Ajdacic-Gross, Ken Arnold, Sarah Bakewell, Margaret Jull Costa, Amelia Crouch, Brian Dillon, Thomas Dixon, Elaine Howard Ecklund, Jules Evans, Gary Foxcroft, Ruth Garde, Michael John Gorman, John Haigh, Will Hammond, Dale Harrow, Emma Hawe, Felicity Henderson, Mark Henderson, Denny Hilton, Philip Hoare, Geoff Hollington, Amanda Ingram, Kevin Killeen, Michael Landy, Stephanie Lichtenfeld, Alison Macfarlane, Robert Macfarlane, Javier Marías, Sheila Marshall, Kris de Meyer, Penny Parks, Graeme Peart, Claire Preston, Elli Resvanis, Stephen Senn, David Spiegelhalter, Anna Waldstein and Marina Warner.

It is regrettably true that Thomas Browne these days has what could politely be described as a select following even among those whose business is words. So I consider myself extremely lucky to have found the ideal publisher for this eccentric project in Granta Books, and my greatest thanks go to Philip Gwyn Jones and my editor there, Max Porter, who walked the walk. I am grateful as well to artists James Nunn and Emily Faccini and to designer Lindsay Nash, for bringing their visual flavour of the seventeenth century, to my copy-editor Martin Bryant, to Christine Lo and Sarah Wasley, who oversaw production, and to Pru Rowlandson and Sara D'Arcy, who rose to the challenge of publicity for my obscure hero. Thanks to Matt Weiland at W. W. Norton for his continued support for my writing. Thanks also to my agent Antony Topping, who made it all happen.

Last, I thank Moira and Sam, who I know won't object if I now go on a bit less about Sir Thomas Browne, physician of Norwich.

Hugh Aldersey-Williams
Norfolk
June 2014

Index

Keep in touch with
Granta Books:

Visit grantabooks.com to discover more.

GRANTA